MEDICAL DISCLAIMER

This publication contains the opinions and ideas of its author. It is intended to provide helpful and informative material on the subjects addressed in the publication. It is sold with the understanding that the author and publisher are not engaged in rendering medical, health, or any other kind of personal professional services in the book. The reader should consult his or her medical, health, or other competent professional before adopting any of the suggestions in this book or drawing inferences from it.

The author and publisher specifically disclaim all responsibility for any liability, loss, or risk, personal or otherwise, that is incurred as a consequence, directly or indirectly, of the use and application of any of the contents of this book.

STARTING
THIS
MONDAY

....

AN *UNCOMPLICATED* GUIDE TO BALANCING FOOD, FITNESS, AND FRIENDS IN JUST FOUR WEEKS

PATTI VANACORE

Vanacore Publishing
MENDHAM, NEW JERSEY

Patti Vanacore / Vanacore Publishing
www.StartingThisMonday.life

Cover design by Gus Yoo
Copy editing and production by Stephanie Gunning
Book Layout © Book Design Templates

Library of Congress Control Number: 2019918778

Starting This Monday / Patti Vanacore. —1st ed.
ISBN 978-0-578-60969-0 (paperback)

CONTENTS

Learn to love what's good for you.

PREFACE

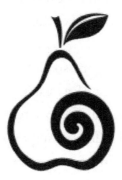

When I had the idea to share my journey to good health with you, I noticed how other health authors seemed to be the epitome of fitness. As a professional fitness trainer for three decades, I am certain that their physiques are nearly unattainable for regular people. When I look at their pictures, it's easy to believe that they have never made mistakes with their diets and have always stayed on course with their fitness routines. I imagine them to have been super-athletes during their high school and college years. I do not want to portray myself like that to you.

One of the reasons I am sharing my weight-loss plan in this book with you is because I get it. I get the struggle to stay the course of wellness. I cannot say that I do everything perfectly every day, and I certainly don't put myself on a pedestal. I make mistakes, I eat crappy on occasion. Some days I just do not want to do it. But nonetheless I am always striving to be "unprocessed" inside and out. Every day. And you can too!

Unprocessed just means that I eat *real* food, instead of packaged food or fast-food, and that most of this wholesome food is made in my home kitchen.

In our society, we have gone so far in our lives beyond meeting our basic needs that many of us can't even remember what the fundamentals are. In general, our society is consumed with buying stuff. We are consumed with working to pay off the debt we have incurred from straining to buy our stuff. We are consumed with getting our kids to the multitude of places they must be. We are busy being busy and, in the process of our busy-ness, we overlook ourselves and fail to grasp what has the power to move us emotionally. We've forgotten to love and honor our bodies. We've stopped buying wholesome, pure, real food because we've stopped having time to cook it. We've stopped going to an exercise group or out for a walk around the block with our dog.

Heck, even our dogs are stressed, overweight, and unhealthy!

We have put off trying that new yoga place downtown because we are taking care of everyone else besides ourselves. We have thought about joining the Meet Up hiking group, but we are afraid we won't be healthy enough to keep up with the other members on the trail or because we do not have enough spare time to make a time commitment.

These things are factors in why people in our society are not as healthy as they could be. It's why we and others we know are not as fit and energized as we would like to be.

I invite you to take a moment right now to notice your breath. Are you breathing smoothly and filling your lungs fully? Or are you shallow breathing, barely expanding your lungs enough to intake any oxygen? If you're like me on days when I forget to slow my roll, then you may be forgetting to take good, deep breaths. Often my shoulders are shrugged up, tightness moves into my neck, and my head starts hurting. Do you ever feel like that?

In everyone's life, there are certain times and events that stand out as significant because they wake us up to what's important. I have experienced several events like this in recent years. I wish that these remarkable events had occurred when I was younger, but there are probably reasons why they didn't happen back then—including the possibility that I simply wasn't paying enough attention because of my busy schedule.

Are you familiar with the adage "When the student is ready, the teacher will appear"? This thought goes back centuries and is as true today as it was when it was first spoken. But it is also true that lessons can be learned everywhere. They surround us. Every moment can teach us a lesson if our minds are present and open enough to see it.

I tell my children to look for lessons every day. The answers are all right there!

A lesson that set me on a new and even better path took place when I went to Italy to celebrate my fiftieth birthday. My nephew was going to college in northern Italy at the time, so I grabbed at the opportunity to meet him in Venice. During this visit, one day he and I had gone to the farmers market to buy some fresh vegetables, cheese, and wine. We stopped at the trattoria outside his apartment. In the piazza, two elderly men were seated at a small table in the warm afternoon sunshine having a passionate conversation about growing grapes for wine. I could tell by their stained hands and weathered faces that they had spent a lifetime making wine. Wine is what moved them. I have this indelible image photographed in my mind as a moment that marked a major shift in my center of being.

Watching these gentlemen taking the time, after a good, hard day of farming their land, to connect with each other to talk about their passion and enjoy a sunny afternoon in the village that they loved was a marker showing me where I was in my own quest for wellbeing. I wanted what they had—a good life where work and leisure were in balance.

I was aware that at some point on my trip a question would be asked in conversation. The question would be, "What do you do?" Italians don't usually ask this because they want to know how people make a living. They want to know who others are and what moves us. But I was dreading this question.

Why was I so nervous to answer it? Because I didn't really know the answer—at least not completely.

It was then that I began to put the puzzle pieces of my good life together back home. It didn't happen overnight. I would spend many years readjusting my "pieces" so they would fit.

A subsequent trip I took to Sedona, Arizona, with a couple of good friends was another experience that changed how I look at things. We had just climbed Cathedral Rock. In fact, we had conquered it! For me, being able to do the rock scramble that is required to get to the top was a triumph as I am afraid of heights. My preconceived notion that the height would be terrifying was exactly that: a preconceived notion. In reality, climbing was an experience that I needed. It was a lesson in perseverance, trusting myself, and working hard for a payoff.

Before we left Sedona, we stopped at a beautiful stream that runs under Cathedral Rock. There were pools of water where the stream gently opened. It was sunset and the amazing spires of the rock face we had just been climbing were reflected in the calm running water. Glints of sunshine accented the towering rocks and illuminated the deep reds of red rock country. I stepped into the pool of water ankle deep, and saw my reflection blending with the reflected spires of Cathedral Rock. In those moments, I realized why I love to be in nature. Nature is my church.

Along the trail under Cathedral Rock people had stopped and taken the time to build towers out of balanced stones of all sizes. It was a meditation in balance. A point in time where time stopped. A place where people had nowhere else to be and nothing else to do except create beauty. The clarity I felt that day looking at those stone towers was transformational.

In order to be able to climb these trails for years to come, I could see that I would need to stay healthy. In order to be able to learn from my surroundings, I could see that my head needed to be clear from the effects of toxic food and toxic people. I had the insight that I needed to eat right and exercise, and make room for positive, happy people and beauty.

Life is about taking the time to balance our stones, whatever they may be. Balance of food, exercise, and the good in life is essential—and that's what you'll get in this book.

INTRODUCTION

STARTING THIS MONDAY

How many times have you said to yourself, "Starting this Monday, I am going on a diet" or "Starting this Monday, I am going to exercise"?

Having the thought in mind that you really need to do something differently—to make some changes—is the first step to implementing positive change.

It is possible that you've thought about this for a while without taking action. Maybe even years.But now you've made a solid move to pick up this plan and start on Monday . . .

For real this time.

The ultimate goal of this four-week plan is overall good health. If you are someone who needs to lose weight that loss *will* come naturally as you progress through these weeks. This plan is not a *diet* in the typical sense of the word. It is a way of eating and exercising that can keep you in balance for the rest of your life.

This plan is a way of incorporating the foods you eat into a lifestyle that is balanced in all of its aspects, including movement and friendship and more. My plan isn't just about not eating the wrong foods and forcing yourself to find some sort of exercise that you like (or can tolerate). It is about finding positivity within yourself and the world surrounding around you, starting with how you treat your inner body.

In no particular order, these are my seven principles for a balanced life.

- **Proper nutrition** Feed your body to feed your soul. Honor and respect your body with nutrient-rich foods from the Earth and plenty of water. Strive for a preservative-free, sugar-free, toxin-free body.
- **Physical activity**. Move your body. I encourage you to find something physical that gets you up and energized.
- **Spend time in nature.** Ecotherapy has been linked to mindfulness, increased creativity, and overall well-being. Being in sunlight—because of the vitamin D it brings—helps prevent seasonal affect disorder (SAD), a condition where people feel blue during the darkness of the winter months.
- **Friendships and relationships.** Connect to others in loving, supportive relationships. Family, friends, clients, animals! A good way to tell if a person is healthy for you is to note the way you feel after being with them. Are they loving and supportive or do you feel exhausted and stressed?
- **Spirituality**. Develop your belief in something greater than yourself, like a god or gods, the power of the Universe, or collective energy. Nature is *my* church.

- **Community service.** Gandhi said, "The best way to find yourself is to lose yourself in the service of others." Filling a portion of your life with service to others or to a specific cause, helps you to connect with others, feel connected, and gives purpose to your own life.

- **Recreation and leisure.** Recreation is doing something you like to do purely for enjoyment. It should refresh you and give you a sense of raised spirits and enthusiasm. For example, you might try music, theater, books, art, culture, and crafts.

Starting new, healthier lifestyle really begins with carefully examining everything you put into your body. Your body is a place of worship; therefore, it should be treated according to this principle what you put into it should be of the highest quality. You should treat it with respect.

Please understand that the reason you may not have been able to let go of your unhealthy food habits in the past (and the extra pounds you may have put on as a result of them) is largely because food is emotionally, and sometimes physically, addictive.

Eliminating unhealthy food, like food filled with sugar or fat, is difficult and requires focus. One of the reasons most diets fail is because they require us to eliminate all unhealthy foods at one time, in one day. These diets also ask that you reduce food intake to the point of great discomfort.

But we don't like discomfort!

Caloric restriction to the point of being constantly hungry does not work. If you're like me, the first four days of a diet are usually OK, but then, on the fifth day, you fall off track. Your body gets hungry and tired and then your mind says, *It's not worth it. I will start again . . . on Monday.*

Most of us have seen (or even tried) diets with no carbs, diets of cabbage or grapefruit and eggs only, and diets where you eat bacon and steak all day long. Most of us have seen diets in books where an author is selling his or her own line of food. And none of these diets work because that way of eating is not at all like eating in real life.

How long could you realistically sustain this sort of plan? You cannot possibly continue for the rest of your life to order food online to be delivered to your doorstep. You cannot possibly eat grapefruit and eggs as your soul food source for the rest of your life.

As humans, we are supposed to eat according to our family of origin. Originally, humans were hunter-gatherers. Depending upon our region, we ate land mammals (including their fat and organs), fish, fowl, eggs, nuts, seeds, plant leaves and stems, insects, fruits, berries, and tubers. Tubers include underground foods, such as carrots, potatoes, sunchokes, and beets, to name only a few. Rice was available in Asia, and in Central America corn was the equivalent staple. And, for the most part, those foods were what people ate to survive. For these reasons these foods are what we are genetically conditioned to eat. Refined grains were introduced much later in the history of civilization.

From an evolutionary perspective, humans have not had the time to genetically change their systems to adapt to all the types of grains we feed ourselves now. I'm not saying to go out and eat an entire animal, and I am not saying that grains are wrong to eat, but in the realm of foods tolerated by the human body, refined grains are not high up on the list. Add to this, that, whatever is available to us has been poisoned for the most part with pesticides. It has been genetically modified. It is grown in nutrient-weak soil. And it is frequently processed to the point of being devalued as a good source of vitamins and minerals.

The amount of poor-quality foods we ingest every day has led to real life-or-death problems in our society. In our society as it is today, it is unusual to find an individual or family who grows their own food, eats entirely organically, cooks meals from "scratch," and basically eats the way their makeup dictates they are supposed to eat. Add to this, with the amount of sugar, salt, and fat consumed every day, you will see that we are following a lifestyle recipe that could be disastrous for your health and well-being. These old dietary habits are hard to break, but with dedication you can discover a much healthier way to survive.

The idea behind *Starting This Monday,* is to replace self-destructive eating behaviors with healthy choices over a four-week period. During these four weeks, you'll also begin to implement an exercise program that you like!

This plan may force you to look at some of the reasons behind why you developed the habits you did. When faced with the questions you will need to ask yourself it may take you to a place of discomfort . As you start looking at some of the reasons why you don't eat healthily or exercise, you may learn some interesting truths about yourself and your upbringing within your family that brought you to this place of being.

So, here's the essence of the plan. By replacing your bad habits with good habits, one moment at a time, every day for four weeks in a row, you will be able to attain a lifestyle that will help you drop weight (if that is your goal) and get a bit more fit—and then bring you more happiness and freedom then than you probably could have imagined. Freedom from food cravings. Freedom from achy joints, fatigue, and energy dips. Happier because you feel in charge of your destiny.

The first step in this plan to imagine yourself as a healthy, strong, and physically independent person. Remember that every choice you make leads to your future outcome.

In your life, you may have developed habits that do not suit your body anymore. Maybe these habits have gotten you to the point that you are sick, tired, and depressed. And you may be ready to make changes, yet you don't know what to do or where to start to get your life and your health on track. You may be holding on to these habits in your adult life for a reason. These habits could be filling an emotional need, or they are habits you learned early in life. Maybe you are now addicted to sugar and white flour, alcohol, or pain medication. This is in part, due to poor eating and exercise habits. The reason you are reading this is because in some way your life is not in balance. It may be a little off or it may be life threatening. My desire in this book is to help you put balance in place over the course of a month so that your path forward from then on is both healthy and fulfilling. Once you've taken these initial few steps.

Deciding to "diet" on Monday and attempting to take all "bad" foods out of your life in one day, and at the same time launching yourself onto a treadmill at top speed will not work. You will burn out or get injured by Thursday.

Changing unhealthy habits and eliminating unhealthy foods is a process that takes time, commitment, and consistency. As you experience positive results and benefit from making changes at a steady, yet reasonable pace, you'll double down on your commitment to them. You'll want to continue this new lifestyle when you learn how good it makes you feel.

Eventually you will realize that honoring your body means eating delicious whole and unprocessed foods, without sugar and white flour. It means being alert to toxic ingredients in your food that you can't see, such as chemical additives.

It also means enjoying an exercise program, one that you like and look forward to. This does not need to cost a lot of money either. Sure, it's important to have a good, sturdy pair of sneakers. But that could be your biggest investment. There are plenty of outdoor activities that are free. Walking is free. Gallon jugs of water cost under a dollar and are refillable—and these can be used as free weights. I will show you how to do a workout with just that equipment.

Tracking is helpful. Journaling about your food intake and exercise helps because of how it makes you more accountable and will help you stop and think before you make a decision to eat something that may be detrimental to your goals.

You may have come to a point in your life where chronic illness and pain have taken over your body. Inflammatory foods like white flour and sugar are causing havoc in your organs. Instead of trying a wholesome approach to anxiety and depression, food and drugs are used first. The lack of fresh air and cardiovascular activity is robbing your body of oxygen and you can see it in the pallor of the skin. You're getting weaker from lack of resistance exercise. Maybe you are losing bone density as well. If you have attempted to change your habits many times and have been unsuccessful, then it's time to do something differently with your approach.

This program can be, will be, a commitment that will not only change how you look and feel, but will help you see how negative eating carries over to negative people and negative behavior choices.

Because you have read this far, you most likely have come to the realization that something has to change. You are now ready to put your research and desire for a better lifestyle into action. Putting thoughts in action will be your first week in *Starting This Monday*. This is something to be proud of. Turn the page and I'll show you how to prepare for Week One.

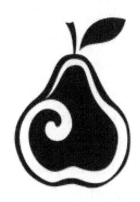

PURGING, SHOPPING, AND MAKING A COMMITMENT

Your body is not a garbage pail, so it's time to stop filling it with garbage.

L ook, You are already ahead! You have considered your options. You have researched the choices. You have already made all your excuses and experienced the results. Now, you've decided not to make excuses anymore. Now you are committed to moving ahead.

The Commitment: Purging Your Pantry

The program I am laying out for you here is founded on several steps of elimination that make room for better choices. As you will see, moving from week to week, this is a gentle shift from one way of living to another.

To prepare to begin this coming Monday by you will need to purge your cabinets and refrigerator of unhealthy sweet foods. You will have one full week to do this! You are starting by purging any added sugar products. This first week of the plan is about getting your head in the game while you are setting up your program for your new and improved way of living. This is all about you—your health and wellbeing—and nothing is more important.

Going forward you will need to purge products containing sugar, white flour, and trans-fat. I suggest you carry this book into your kitchen and do that right now! I would like to see you completely clean out all foods that contain these three elements.

Later on, you will be able to add back, in moderation, some of the foods you are purging now, but not yet. We are going to assume, for the duration of this program, that you need to avoid sugar and white flour entirely because you are addicted to them. This program is relying on you to stay the course.

This cleanout should include all bread made with sugar, salad dressings, snack foods, ketchup, crackers, and cookies. Yogurt that is not "plain," coffee creamers, frozen products, and processed foods, to name a few items. And don't forget soda. Also, diet products with fake sugar (saccharine, aspartame, and so on) need to go. You've got to get used to discovering the flavor of whole, real foods. Your body, and that includes your brain, needs to become accustomed to the taste of foods without sweeteners. Over these four weeks, you'll be rediscovering the flavor of whole, real foods.

Read every label. Even if you think there is no sugar added, read the label anyway. You probably will be surprised where sugar hides. I was! Every single bit of product with added sugar, white flour, and trans-fat has to go in the garbage.

Think about this fact when you look at sugar grams on the label: Every sixteen grams of sugar equals four teaspoons of sugar.

Please don't make excuses about throwing food away. Do not tell me that this action is wasteful. **Your body is not a garbage pail**. If you feel terrible about getting rid of food, then donate it to a food bank if you can. Check the expiration date though. Don't "save it for the kids," as your kids do not need to have a sugar overload either. Unless they are in competitive sports or are vigorously exercising for a least one hour every day, they should not be consuming sugar or any of the other products I mentioned! All you are doing if you let them eat that way is setting them up to be sugar addicts and poor eaters later in life.

Starting this coming Monday and for the rest of this week, you will be looking for healthy options for your breakfast, lunch, snacks, and dinner. By purging your kitchen and taking away all temptations, you will be setting yourself up for success. Don't try to tell yourself that you won't eat this or that because you are in charge. That is like putting alcohol in front of an alcoholic. Whether or not you want to admit it, if you ever tried to take sugar (and flour) out of your diet before and failed, then you are addicted to them.

Believe me, I understand that this is a strong statement and that it is difficult to look at eating food in this way. But blood sugar spikes, whether or not you feel them, are the main reason why diets fail and why this plan has to be done in steps.

Keep in mind, this changing habits takes time and dedication. There is no quick fix, no instant gratification when it comes to losing weight. But your energy and cravings for sugar and flour should stabilize in the first week once they are out of your diet. Stay the course. Throughout the upcoming week, to really dig in and stop putting sugar into your body may be a challenge initially. Stay committed!

The idea is to keep your blood sugar stable throughout the day. If your blood sugar gets low, you will get hungry and crave unhealthy foods that contain sugar. The go-to for most people when a craving hits is a candy bar—or a sugar-laden bar that says "healthy" on its label. Terrible choices because they keep you addicted to sweets. The other go-to your body will crave will most likely be something like crackers or chips. Another not-great choice.

This is why small frequent meals are imperative. Don't let yourself get hungry. To do this, you will eat every three hours. Depending on when you start your day the basic rule is breakfast, snack, lunch, snack, and a light dinner.

Learn to know the difference between hunger, frustration, boredom, and other emotional triggers. Also learn to know the difference between thirst and hunger. Keep hydrated.

—Hydration Tip—

You should be drinking .66 ounces of water per day per pound of body weight. For a 125-pound person that means 82.5 ounces. For a 185-pound person that means 122.1 ounces.

To calculate your approximate water intake, multiply your weight x 66 percent. For example, let's say you weigh 155 pounds. Multiply 155 x .66 = 102.3. That would be 102.3 in ounces!

Now that you have your cabinets cleaned out, it's time to go shopping. Purchase fresh fruits to help with your soon-to-be sugar cravings. You may replace every sugar craving with a small helping of fresh fruit. Have the fruit already cut up. Purchase crunchy veggies, such as celery, carrots, and cucumbers. Cut these up and have them ready in the fridge.

This week coming up you are only removing added sugar from your food. If you need the satisfaction of crackers or chips to get you through your cravings during this first program week, it is acceptable. Be moderate in your consumption, however. Remember the rule to check the label of everything you buy, looking for added sugar. Don't bring anything into the house that deviates from the plan.

Why risk it?

In Week One, you will need to keep your protein level high. This will help slow down the process of digestion and stabilize your blood sugar level.

Your Basic Shopping List: Foundation of a Healthy Kitchen

Here is a basic shopping list that will ensure you have healthy food in your cabinets and refrigerator on the first day of Week One.

Fresh Produce:
All fresh vegetables and leafy greens
All fresh fruits
Yams/sweet potatoes
Leeks, onions, scallions, and other roots

Meat/Fish Protein:
Fish, especially salmon, tuna, and white fish
Game, such as buffalo and venison
Chicken, white meat
Turkey, white meat
Lean red meat
Pork

Grains:

Brown or black rice

Whole-grain bread (but check the label, and say no to added sugar)

Whole-grain wraps

Oatmeal, amaranth, quinoa, faro, kamut, or other hot grain cereals

Legumes:

Kidney beans

Black beans

Garbanzo beans (aka chickpeas)

Pinto beans

All beans are acceptable

Nuts and Seeds:

Raw almonds, cashews, macadamias, pecans, walnuts

Sunflower seeds

Pumpkin seeds

Peanut butter

Almond butter

Dairy:

Low-fat string cheese

Plain low-fat yogurt (Greek or Scandinavian)

Low-fat milk/unsweetened almond milk

Eggs and egg whites

Staples:

Extra-virgin olive oil

Sesame oil

Balsamic vinegar

Lemon

Condiments and spices

Tea

Coffee

Bottled water (if your home doesn't have a filter on the kitchen tap)

Getting Your Head on Straight: Make the Commitment

Exercise and food preparation are appointments you must make with yourself to succeed in this program. This is all about getting ready emotionally and logistically. Making a verbal commitment to yourself and the people around you is important. Figuring out when, where, and how you are going to eat is also vital to your success. Don't wing it. You're setting yourself up for failure unless you think it through.

You will need to eat every three hours. Where will you be sourcing your food from? While writing your shopping list think about your week and plan for every single meal.

Another commitment you'll be making is to do twenty minutes of exercise every day. Starting on Monday, be ready to go with this component of your new life of balance and good health. These components of food and exercise must go hand in hand if you want your program to be successful.

What are you doing during your day that could be modified to make room for some healthy activity? Is it possible to give up twenty minutes of social media chatting or watching television? I always tell my clients that if they have time for social media and television, then they have time to get some exercise. Even if it means setting your alarm to get up twenty minutes earlier in the morning, it will be worth it. Or maybe make a quick twenty-minute stop at a park for a walk or jog before you head home. This will give you a chance to unwind and decompress. If it means life or death—and your health does—then you will find a way.

WEEK ONE

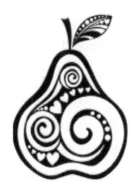

SAY GOODBYE TO ADDED SUGAR

Say these words if you feel pressured: "I am committed to living a healthier life."

Starting this Monday, today, you are going to say goodbye to all *added* sugar. As opposed to the natural sugar that is found in fruits, vegetables, and dairy. Here is why. An average American eats 130 pounds of added sugar a year. If you eat too much sugar, your pancreas must work overtime producing insulin to process the over-abundance. Insulin is a hormone made by the pancreas that allows the body to gradually process the carbohydrates you consume. When the pancreas has to work extra hard over a long period of time, the tissue of the organ eventually breaks down. When it is finally exhausted and broken after all the sugar consumption, you become a diabetic. That is an overly simplified explanation, of course.

There are several types of diabetes. For our purpose, what you should be aware of is type 2 diabetes. Type 2 is the most common form of this disease. To date. there are 29.1 million cases in the United States, and as many as 8.1 million people may be undiagnosed. Genetic factors, inactivity, and poor nutrition may contribute to the development of type 2 diabetes. This form of the disease used to be known as adult-onset diabetes. But since more children are being diagnosed with it, most likely due to the rise in childhood obesity, the original name has been dropped. Losing weight, eating healthfully, and exercising, as well as possibly taking medication, if a medical doctor prescribes it, is the way to control the symptoms of the disease.[1]

Beyond diabetes, many more health issues arise from the overconsumption of sugar. These include obesity, inflammation of the heart and organs, inflammation of the joints, excessive yeast growth, and mood swings.

Sugar is also addictive. The way your system reacts to sugar is very much like the way your system reacts to opioids and many other addictive drugs. Once ingested, your body is stimulated to release dopamine, a hormone and neurotransmitter that makes you feel good. It's the exact same hormone that is released when we ingest cigarettes, heroin, cocaine, and other addictive drugs. After your dopamine level drops again, you may notice that you're feeling crummy and your body will signal that it wants more with cravings. Because of this, sugar is hard to give up.

The cravings when you say goodbye to added sugar can be intense. Don't be surprised if you feel sick, even possibly running a low-grade fever along with experiencing joint aches and pain. You may also have a headache, feel nauseous, and feel anxiety, anger, or irritability. These are symptoms of the detox process. Push through it. It takes a lot of willpower.

Also be gentle with yourself. The week you give up sugar isn't the week to make a lot of plans and put yourself under pressure. Do your best to stay relaxed. Drink lots of water to flush the remaining sugar out of your body. In a few days, you'll feel better.

What to Expect When You Give Up Added Sugar This Week

Giving up sugar is a process that is very much the same as giving up drug addiction. It is a universal process that happens in steps. What I am saying is that you are not alone. Almost everyone who has gone through a detox or is in the midst of giving up one or more of their vices goes through the ups and downs of detox.

The first step is making the decision (and summoning the motivation) to give up the habit!

A day or so after quitting sugar, you will likely begin to have cravings for sweet things. These craving typically last from one to seven days; the duration depends on how much sugar an individual has been consuming until then. This is the period when your mind will start to battle with you. It may say, "Hey, you really don't need to do this," "Listen, you can have just one cookie," or "You are *not* a sugar addict. I can't believe you're doing this to me!"

Ignore those voices and carry on!

Respond to the cravings by doing some exercise or having a piece of fruit and some protein.

Refined sugar offers you no nutritional value to speak of; however, when you eat fruit or vegetables, you are nourishing your body with vital nutrients, fiber, and energy.

After the cravings start, you may think you have caught a cold or flu. I have had clients who have said to me, "I am eating all this healthy food, and I am exercising, but now I am sick!" You are not sick, you are detoxing. Drink lots of water and eat fruit and protein. Rest as much as possible. Soon you will start feeling better. Look forward to that day.

Keep positive. Imagine yourself strong and well. Picture what your future will look like when you have balance and good health.

And finally, you will feel clear headed and energetic.

Stick with it. Ride the waves of emotions and cravings. Remember that this detox is not going to last forever. This is a temporary commitment because you have chosen to live a healthy life. At some point you will be able to add some of these forbidden foods back into your life, but for now, stay on track.

Going forward this week, it's going to get tricky. This is when you learn it's not only a physical challenge to stop eating refined sugar, it's emotional too. Sugar addiction is real.

Be ready to turn down some social situations this week and keep your routines simple. This week is crucial to the rest of your life. So, if avoiding sugar means hunkering down and staying in until you are confident in your food choices, then you should do it. If you can, suggest your social occasion is to meet in a park and go for a walk rather than dining together.

I understand that occasionally your schedule will not allow for this: For example, sometimes we have to attend business meetings that require us to be around food or you are obliged to attend a family event such as a wedding or child's birthday party. You may find yourself having to go out to eat because of social or work demands. If that is the case, then look at it this way: Ordering a healthy meal sets a good example for your friends and coworkers.

I mentioned earlier that going to a restaurant when you are hungry is not the best plan of action.

I suggest that you have a snack that contains approximately one hundred calories before you go. I suggest the one hundred-calorie snack packs of nuts that many stores sell these days, a piece of string cheese, a hardboiled egg, or a spoonful of peanut butter or almond butter. If you consume about one hundred calories, it will help to ward off hunger pangs. These calories ideally should contain protein as this will help to curb your appetite for a couple hours.

Check the ingredient label. The nuts you purchase should be *raw*. Oil should not be mentioned. And regarding nut butters (peanut butter and almond butter, for example), be sure yours does not contain other types of oils or sugar.

- Research eating establishments before you eat out. Know what you will be ordering from the menu. Immediately ask for a salad with balsamic dressing and water or seltzer with lemon.
- This week you are only eliminating added sugar. I begrudgingly will say that pasta is allowed; however, be moderate with carbs!
- Choose a meal that is not creamy or buttery because you don't know what is actually in the sauce. Many times, the sauce contains added sugar.
- The rule is that if you can't identify the ingredients you must stay away from it.

Although four weeks of eating clean, sugar-free food could seem like a long time, picture it day by day. Keep imagining yourself as a strong and healthy person, a person who wants a healthy and balanced life. Every night before you go to sleep, imagine what your future will look like. Wake up every morning with the same attitude.

As the first week progresses, expect your body and mind to try to trick you into thinking that you never meant to sign up for this challenge. Your mind is probably going to say, "Hey, someone brought donuts to work, you should have one to be polite." Or it may say, "You are not a sugar addict, so you can skip this part."

Ignore those types of thoughts. That's the sugar talking.

If you don't feel ill the first day or so, that's great. But keep up your guard because you could still start having symptoms. Days four and five are typically the most difficult for my training clients when I give them this eating plan to follow, for the reasons we've previously discussed.

Use your will power and have faith in yourself that at the end of this week you will have accomplished a sugar detox.

Stay the course and don't be tempted. You have to want this more than anything!

Actions for Week One

Over the weekend, to prepare yourself for this four-week program, you put healthy food choices in place. You cleaned out your fridge and cabinets and went shopping, so everything you have on hand right now is fresh. There should not be any moldy produce in the crisper drawer. There should be no expired food packages.

From now on, you will respect the food that you are bringing into your home and putting in your body. This food is nourishing you with wellness.

Continue to read all labels searching for added sugar. Some other names for sugar are high-fructose corn syrup, cane sugar, brown sugar syrup, molasses, sucrose, monosaccharides, honey, and "natural" sugar (really, food manufacturers try to trick us).

Be aware that sugar is often added into bread, soups, salad dressings, tomato sauce, cereals, canned vegetables, and yogurt to name only a few products.

Throw ALL these products away when you find them in your house. Yes, really.

A Note about Artificial Sweeteners

Stay away from artificial sweeteners. Right now, I want your brain and taste buds to get used to the taste and positive effects of whole (real) food. Both Andrew Weil, M.D., and Mehmet Oz, M.D., suggest that we not consume these products.[2] Dr. Oz says: "Sweeteners, which can be 300 times sweeter than natural sugar, are known to increase appetite and result in overeating. Be on the lookout for artificial sweeteners, and when possible, steer clear of them."[3]

Artificial sweeteners are an ingredient to search for when you are reading labels. Although the FDA says there is no risk to humans in eating these products, here are some scientific claims being made against artificial sweeteners, which are notably found in diet sodas and diet drinks.

- A Dutch study showed that the risk of premature births increased 78 percent among women who drank four or more diet sodas per day.[4]

- A Harvard University study showed that the habit of drinking two or more diet sodas per day is associated with kidney function decline.[5]
- A study jointly conducted by researchers from Columbia University and the University of Miami found a 43 percent increased risk of heart attack and stroke among those who consumed diet soda.[6]
- An association has been found between artificial sweeteners and headaches, diarrhea, cramps, and yeast infections.[7]
- The Medical College of Wisconsin did a study linking artificial sweeteners to diabetes and obesity. The claim is that these sweeteners change the way the body processes fat.[8]

That's why you need to say goodbye to artificial sweeteners along with added sugar.

The Importance of Exercising When You're Quitting Sugar

Exercising is a good substitute for eating sugar. It replaces negative behavior with something positive. And it raises your dopamine level, making you feel happier. That is why it is imperative that you start your exercise program today. Interestingly, exercise also raises energy levels. So, if you're feeling mopey while quitting sugar, it will give you a lift.

This week, find twenty minutes every day to break a sweat. This should be part of your daily schedule and should be treated as an important meeting. It is a meeting with your body to get yourself to the place you want to be in life.

You don't need to join a gym or publicly exercise if you are not ready. Simply move your body. Do a few rounds of sit-ups, stretching in between; follow along with a yoga class on YouTube or an exercise program on TV; or lace up your sneakers and go for a walk.

Here is a Water Jug Workout that you can do at home.

The Water Jug Workout

For this workout routine, you will need a sealable jug with a handle on it that you can grip, which holds a gallon of water. You can control the weight by how full you keep the jug.

¼ gallon of water = 2.8 pounds
½ gallon of water = 4.17 pounds
1 gallon of water = 8.34 pounds

If a gallon (eight pounds) seems heavy to you, you can start by pouring out some of the water (drink it or use it to water your plants). As you gain strength, fill the jug with more water.

Exercise 1. Strengthen Your Biceps (Curls)

You'll begin with some biceps curls.

1. With one hand, hold the jug by the handle, thumb facing up. (See photo below.)
2. Bend your arm, keeping your elbow hinged to your side. (See photo on the next page.)
3. Return to the starting position.
4. Do ten repetitions.
5. Switch to the opposite arm and repeat.

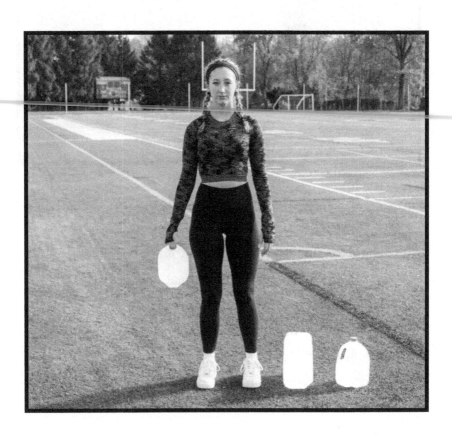

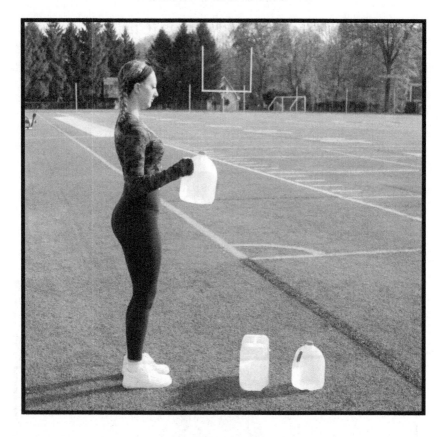

Exercise 2. Strengthen Your Triceps (Curls)

Use a chair for this exercise. (See photos next page.)

1. Place one hand on the chair seat and bend at the waist. Use your other hand to hold the jug, palm facing your torso.
2. Keeping your elbow hinged to your side, drop your forearm to a 45-degree angle.
3. Now extend your arm fully back so it's straight behind you.
4. Bend your arm back to starting position.

5. Do ten repetitions.
6. Switch arms and repeat the sequence.

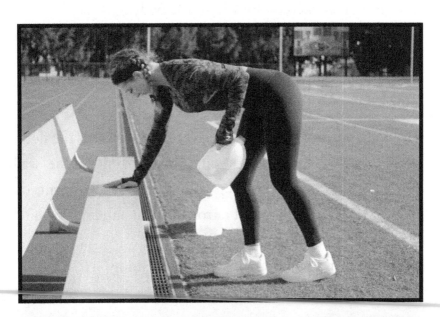

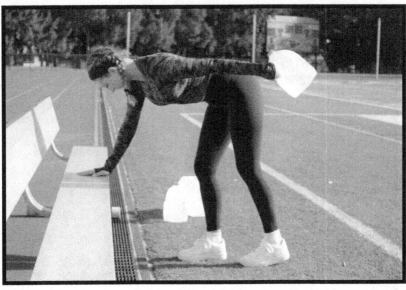

Exercise 3. Strengthen Your Legs (Squats)

This is a great exercise for the whole body.

1. Hold the jug with both hands. Stand tall with your feet hip-width apart. Toes are pointing forward. Position the weight of your body on your heels. (See photos below and on the next page.)

2. Bend your knees and sink your hips towards the floor. As you squat, keep your hips moving to the wall behind you. Also keep your knees in alignment; do not let them bow out or roll in. Your shoulders should be back and your gaze slightly up.

3. Return to an upright standing position.

4. Repeat ten times.

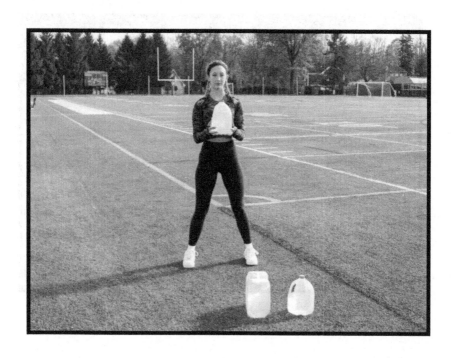

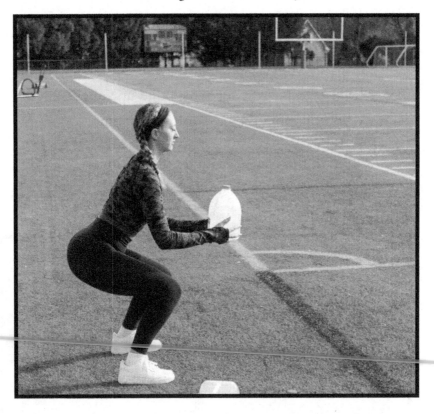

Exercise 4. Strengthen Your Upper Body (Planks)

This one is excellent for maintaining good posture.

1. Begin on your hands and knees with hands directly under the shoulders.
2. Turn your toes under and move your feet back so that your knees come off the floor and your legs are straight behind you. In this "plank" position, your shoulders and hips will form a straight line. (See photo on the next page.)Pull in your abdominal muscles. Do not let your hips either sink or lift. Look

slightly ahead on the floor and keep your neck long. In a correctly neutral position, you will not be dropping your head or lifting your chin.

3. Begin with 15 or 30 seconds. Build up your strength so you can hold the pose for a full minute.

Modification: If the plank position puts too much pressure on your wrists, then move onto your elbows.

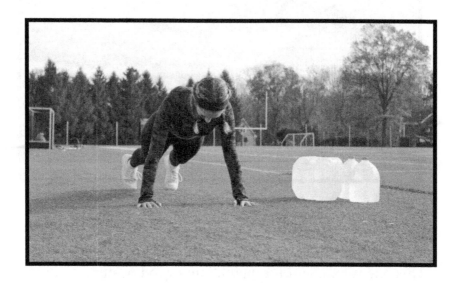

Exercise 5. Strengthen Your Back (Single-Arm Row)

Use a chair for this exercise.

1. Place one hand on the seat of the chair and bend at the waist. Holding a water jug in your other hand, let it hang towards the floor. Your palm should be facing in towards your torso. Your back should be flat. (See photo below.)
2. Pull the jug up to your hip, bending the elbow but keeping the elbow close to your body as it moves up towards your hip. (See photo on the next page.)
3. Return to the starting position.
4. Do ten repetitions.
5. Switch arms and repeat the sequence on other side.

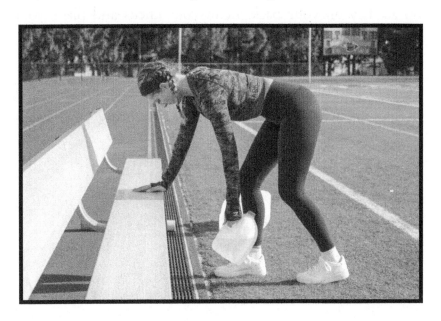

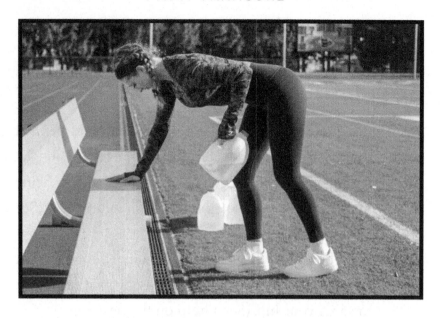

Exercise 6. Strengthen Your Abdominals (Crunches)

This is beneficial for the core.

1. Lay on your back. Bend your knees and place your hands behind your head to support it. (See photos on the next page.)

2. Gently lift your upper body off the ground keeping your chin up. At the same time, bring your knees towards your chest.

3. Repeat ten times.

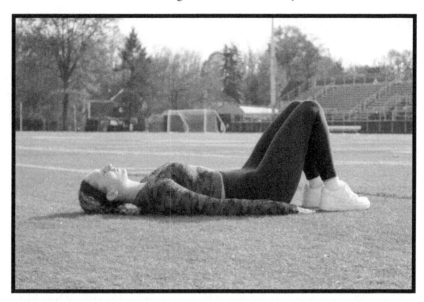

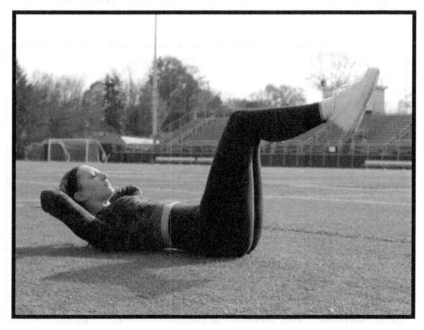

Exercise 7. Stretches

This should feel delicious for your low back and butt.

1. Lay on your back. Bring your knees towards your chest. Keep your lower back on the floor (don't roll up).
2. Cross one shin over the opposite thigh.
3. Gently push the top leg away from you by pressing lightly above your knee. You will feel a stretch in your hip, glute, and low back.
4. Hold the stretch for twenty seconds or longer.
5. Switch legs and repeat the sequence on the other side.

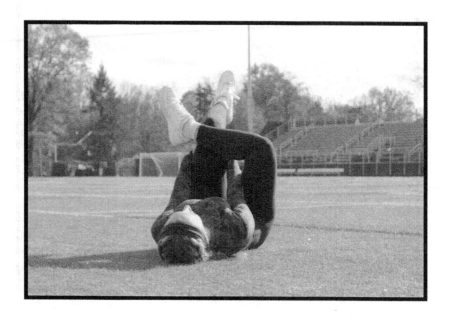

Getting Ready for Week Two

As you are nearing the end of Week One and the elimination of sugar, you should begin writing your food shopping list for Week Two. Going into Week Two, you will go further by taking added sugars and white flour out of your menu. Permutations of white flour include, but are not limited to, baked goods and products like pizza, bagels, pasta, crackers, cereals, chips, and bread.

Go back to your grocery list and replace any items like bread and pasta on it with brown rice, yams, baked potato, legumes, or grains that do not contain white flour. Don't forget to stock up on lots of fresh vegetables and fruits. As you learned last week, read the ingredient labels carefully for surprises. For example, whole-wheat bread very often contains white flour.

Other names for white flour are enriched flour, all-purpose flour, and enriched wheat flour. You're better off with whole-*grain* bread (as opposed to whole-*wheat*). Note the difference and read the ingredient label before bringing home a product anyway.

Look at your schedule for the coming week. Note when you might need to pack food to go. Never leave the house without planning ahead. If you are going to be gone for more than a few hours, bring a healthy snack with you. You need resources when you're feeling hungry.

In addition to planning your food choices, be sure to write down on your weekly schedule exactly when you will exercise. Remember that exercise is an appointment you make with yourself. Enter the days and times into your calendar that you intend to exercise this week.

Week Two will be a great week. You will start to understand and learn additional new habits. Now that you are off sugar, your brain will begin to think clearly and in a positive direction instead of trying to play games with you. Stay strong and focused. You've got this!

WEEK ONE
EXERCISE & NUTRITION
JOURNAL

WEEK TWO

THE NEGATIVE EFFECTS OF WHITE FLOUR

Your body is a temple. Worship it.

Here we are in Week Two. Time to take out the white flour products!

Why is white flour bad for you? White flour products are the result of harvesting wheat berries, and then removing the bran and germ, which are the parts of the berry that are the most nutritious. When removing these two elements, at least fifteen healthy nutrients are removed. Bran is a fiber that is crucial for digestion. Without proper digestion, you will feel bloated and your intestines will get backed up, causing inflammation in your organs. Your colon will become like a toxic waste dump, making it a landscape that promotes colon cancer and other serious ailments.

Why else? White flour digests way too quickly, and this causes an insulin spike, just like when you consume more sugar than your body can handle. The level of your blood sugar (aka glucose) rises and then dramatically decreases, making you feel ravenously hungry again—especially for carbohydrates. This surging is an attack on the body that leads to weight gain, food cravings, lethargy, diabetes, brain fog, and a number of other symptoms and conditions.

Studies also have shown that consuming white flour products contributes to a higher percentage of belly fat. It all goes back to the insulin spikes. When you eat carbs in excess, your body stores molecules it cannot use quickly as fat. Very often, this fat—the fat that comes from too much insulin in the bloodstream—is stored both *viscerally* (between and around your organs) and *subcutaneously* (under your skin). This causes you to end up overweight or obese.

These phenomena, combined with the fact that the bleaching process of flour is toxic, is why consumption of white flour leads to overall horrible health.

A Quick Read about the History of White Flour

White flour used to be aged with time—it took about twelve weeks! This slow process improved the proteins and gluten in the flour, which were great qualities for baking.[1] Around 1900, people decided they wanted their flour whiter.

Consumers no longer liked the natural yellowish appearance of their flour. They wanted "clean-looking" flour, so the bleaching process was introduced. This new way of processing flour was better for manufacturers who could produce it in only forty-eight hours. Ever since then, peroxide agents—most commonly benzoyl peroxide—have been used to whiten the flour. This same chemical is used in topical acne medications with warnings on their product labels from the FDA stating that even topical use may cause severe reactions.[2] Another chemical used to accelerate the process of making white flour whiter was potassium bromate. This is a concern, since scientists have linked bromate use in baking to cancer in lab animals.[3] Instead of banning bromates, as many other countries have done, thus far the FDA has only encouraged bakers to stop using it voluntarily.[4]

Chemist Harvey Washington Wiley, M.D., born in 1844, was a strong advocate for unadulterated food and drugs. He dedicated his life to protecting the public, continually legislating for the safe manufacturing of food and drugs. In the late 1800s, Dr. Wiley was appointed chemist to the U.S. Department of Agriculture. His job was to develop analytical methods to investigate the properties of fertilizers, dairy products, honey, spices, and alcoholic beverages. Because of the extensive research by Dr. Wiley and his team of advocates and activists, known as the Poison Squad, the Pure Food and Drugs Act of 1906 was passed and signed into law by president Theodore Roosevelt. This legislation, promoted to Congress by Dr. Wiley, was the first to address mislabeling of foods and drugs. The law also prohibited the addition of additives that would substitute for food (such as sawdust and other fillers). The Pure Food and Drug Act was passed to protect consumers from dangerous contaminants, such as dirt, fungus, stones, and animal droppings.[5]

In her book *The Poison Squad*, Pulitzer Prize-winning author Deborah Blum tells the true story of the methodical testing of foods processed with harmful additives and dangerous compounds. One of these tests was done on the manufacturing of white bread. In 1910, Dr. Wiley took a case against manufacturers using the bleaching process all the way to the U.S. Supreme Court. Although the case was won—the courts deemed bleaching or altering flour in any way was unlawful—the laws were never enforced. The battles in courts for fair and honest marketing continue to this day.[6]

Be aware that the process for the production of white flour has not substantially changed since the invention of the mill. Bromates and bleach are still used, which is why from now on you are going to be exclusively eating whole-grain bread.

Gluten

When eaten in moderation, gluten is not harmful. Although some people are allergic to it, it is well tolerated by most of us and does not cause inflammation. Gluten is a natural protein found in popular grains, such as wheat, barley, rye, bulger, couscous, and semolina. Many processed products contain it. Here are a few to note: broth, soy sauce, seasonings, and condiments.

Why should we be concerned about gluten? Over time, due to genetic modifications and mutations, the structure of wheat has changed. Today it can possibly contribute to overall inflammation in the body.

If eating wheat upsets your stomach or digestive tract, it is possible that you have a gluten sensitivity. The symptoms of this condition include bloating, diarrhea, and/or constipation, headache, and skin conditions. A good way to determine if you are sensitive to gluten is to take it completely out of your diet for a few weeks. Reintroduce it after this period and see how you feel.

It is also possible that you have irritable bowel syndrome (IBS) if you have abdominal cramping and diarrhea. Very often, but not always, IBS is stress related.

What I am really saying is this: If you have digestive symptoms, you must be your own advocate. Research your symptoms, assess the features of your daily diet, and then ask yourself whether there is anything that could be triggering the symptoms you have.

Another possibility is that you have celiac disease. The only way to diagnose celiac is to have your doctor run a blood test. Celiac disease is a genetic condition, and therefore irreversible. If you have it, you can control the symptoms, but you will always have the disease. Be aware of being misdiagnosed. Celiac disease is an autoimmune disease that can cause severe damage to the intestinal tract. There is no clear reason why celiac disease is on the rise. Some research points to genetics, some to the overuse of antibiotics, some to the *hygiene hypothesis,* which, to put it simply, says that the contemporary lack of exposure to germs makes us susceptible to toxins found in modern wheat.[7]

My own belief is that we simply eat too much wheat and this, when it is combined with multiple other factors, can lead to overall inflammation and damage to your body.

Gliadin

A second important component of wheat is *gliadin.* Along with gluten, it is the primary protein in wheat. However, the present-day gliadin has been compromised due to decades of agricultural production. Scientists have grafted wheat with other types of grass. They induced the mutation of wheat seeds and germ with x-rays and chemicals.[8]

According to cardiologist William Davis, M.D., cardiologist and author of *Wheat Belly,* gliadin was crucially changed due to this process. Dr. Davis claims that this protein breaks down and eventually binds to the opiate receptors of your brain. The desire to eat more of it leads to an addiction to wheat products, and to withdrawal symptoms when you can't get it which are similar to those you experience when you quit sugar.[9]

Glyphosate

Glyphosate, a weed killer and crop desiccant commonly used by farmers in the United States, is now understood to be toxic. A reliable study shows that its presence in our food supply contributes to the destruction of the intestinal tract. This product is routinely sprayed on crops to prevent weeds from mixing in with them and right before harvest, so the unharvested plants dry up quickly, making it easier to plow under the fields and prepare them for the next planting.[10]

Every year, nonorganic farmers dump millions of pounds of glyphosate on crops intended for humans and for animals that are consumed by humans. The fields in which these crops are grown are also grazing areas for wild animals. These levels of glyphosates are so high that federal scientists have detected weed killer in rain and air. Pesticide-exposure scientist Warren Porter, Ph.D., professor of environmental toxicology and zoology at the University of Wisconsin, revealed exposure to this chemical could potentially alter your hormones, leading to obesity, heart problems and diabetes.[11]

Let me just say that if you can buy foods without glyphosate contamination, you may be doing yourself and your family a huge favor. As of this writing, the jury is still out on this product. California's environmental protection agency declared this product a probable carcinogen. Bayer Corporation, who bought Monsanto, the company that produces Roundup, a controversial glyphosate-based herbicide, has had thousands of lawsuits filed against them to date. These claimants say that the herbicide has caused cancer. Among the cases that have gone to trial is the case of a couple who won $2 billion. Both of them became ill with non-Hodgkin's lymphoma after using Roundup on their property for decades. A school groundskeeper who claimed Roundup caused non-Hodgkin lymphoma won $80 million.[12]

I believe it is no coincidence that the significant rise in gut issues, including celiac, IBS, and gluten sensitivity, corresponds with the amount of glyphosate and other herbicides (weed/plant killers) sprayed on the produce that we consume on a daily basis.

I encourage you to never use this product glyphosate (Roundup) in your own farming. If you are growing your own food, there are many ways of preventing weeds from taking over your garden. If you haven't ventured into the realm of gardening, or even of planting some planters with veggies, it is a rewarding way of life—a very nice hobby. Regardless, do not use pesticides.

Buy organic fruits and vegetables whenever possible. The price of organic produce is coming down, as more and more farmers and farming corporations are going organic. Be mindful of the meat you purchase as well, as the lands where animals graze may have been sprayed extensively with glyphosate or the animals may have been fed feed.

Genetically Modified Organisms (GMOs)

Many plants, animals, and other species (for example, bacteria and fungi) have had their genetic makeup altered in a laboratory by humans. Why is this bad? Critics say genetic modification disturbs the genetic code and may possibly cause toxic or allergenic organisms and reactions. I might add that, as of this date, countries that have banned GMOs include France, Germany, Austria, Hungary, Poland, Greece, Luxembourg, and China.[13]

Week Two Actions

Hopefully you have gotten your food shopping done and are ready to forge ahead through the second week. Whole grains in modification, please! Taking white flour out of your diet will be a challenge for you if you are used to eating cereal for breakfast, sandwiches for lunch, and bread or pasta with dinner. Starting with breakfast time, scrambled eggs or frittatas stuffed with veggies are a great start to your day. If you are in a hurry, try plain yogurt with fruit. If you hate yogurt, try a hardboiled egg with fruit. Unless you have managed to locate a sugar-free cereal, this food product has already been eliminated in Week One.

Yes, cereal is quick and easy for you and your kids, but there are many things wrong with it. For example:

1. Most packaged cereals contain sugar and over processed grain.

2. It won't sustain you very long, and you will end up being hungry.

3. There isn't enough protein in it to sustain you for very long.

Changing how you eat will take some time and creativity. I understand that the new food doesn't taste the same as the old food, but you have conditioned yourself to not like "this kind of food" so now you need to change your habits and perceptions. Gradually, you will get used to the taste of simple foods made with minimal ingredients. Remind yourself that this process is a lifestyle change.

Here are a few more tips for you for Week Two.

- Remember, if you are going to a restaurant, you must know before you go. Have an idea of what you are going to order before you get to the destination. Go online and look at the menu, but don't bother to read the pasta selections. You're NOT going to eat pasta.

- If you're going to have a carbohydrate dish at meals, such as bread, potatoes, or rice, plan on having only one serving. For example, do not have both a roll and a baked potato. It's either/or.

- Instead of bread to make a sandwich, use romaine lettuce.

- Instead of crackers for a dip, use cucumber slices or sticks.

- Keep eating veggies and fruit.

- Keep eating plain yogurt and nuts.
- Enjoy lots of salads with grilled chicken, lean meat, or fish accompanying them and dressed with homemade balsamic and olive oil dressing.
- Switch from white rice to brown rice or black rice, yam, or baked potato.
- Make a big pot of lentil soup, chili, or veggie soup with chicken, and always have it on hand.

Remember to eat every three hours (to stabilize your blood sugar) and move your body every day for at least twenty minutes. No exceptions!

Surround Yourself with Positive People

You are the captain of your ship, so you get
to choose who you let on your boat.

We have been discussing toxic foods, but toxic people and toxic work environments can be a problem too. Dieting takes an emotional toll on everybody who diets, which is why you must be on the alert so you can avoid temptation. It is important to keep in mind that sometimes the people around you do not always have your best interest at heart. For reasons of their own, they will try to sabotage your quest for health. You may come across toxic people in your workplace. Likewise, sometimes your friends will want you to partake in their bad habits. You also may find that your family becomes angry at you because they don't understand what you are trying to do. I stress the importance of staying on track no matter how other people react to your choices.

People, especially those you are in relationship with, can feel threatened by your new lifestyle. They may be afraid that you won't be the same person as you were before. It may be painful to admit, but maybe you won't be the same person after you change some of your bad habits.

If a marriage or romance has been built on sharing unhealthy habits and you give them up though your partner doesn't, then you will need to search your soul to decide how to be with this person.

People may try to sabotage your quest for good health out of jealousy. They may need to change their own habits and yet feel unable to commit to a healthier diet and exercise program of their own. But I have found that asking directly for support often works with both friends and family.

It's important to surround yourself with people on the same path as you. Consider joining a support group or a walking club. Most of all, however, you need to rely on your own inner strength and motivation. Your efforts to get healthier are ultimately about you, and nobody else. You cannot change another person's path in life, just like nobody can change yours. It is important to stay firm with your commitment. Saying this line when you're being tested can be a lifesaver. *"I am committed to healthy eating and exercise."*

Remember this: If you choose to stay on the path you were on, you would have become ill. A life-threatening disease would have eventually caught up to you.

Are You an Emotional Eater?

Be honest with yourself. If you truly want to be healthy, to feel energized, to exercise on a regular schedule, and to live a clean and vibrant life, what is holding you back? This is the time, if you have not done it, to say to yourself "I am eating because I am _____ (lonely, bored, angry, ashamed, and so forth—whatever is true for you)." And in place of eating unhealthy food or too much food, to decide "I am going to replace this food with _____."

No doubt you've heard of how eating habits can change in response to intense emotions, such as stress, loneliness, anger, sadness, or boredom. Typically, this type of eating is referred to as *emotional eating*.

Keep in mind, however, that positive emotions could affect your eating choices as much as negative emotions. For example, when a big business deal has been signed, it can be followed by a toast with an alcohol beverage accompanied by a big steak and french fries. Expectations and desire for this type of reward very often are put in place as a child when your parents rewarded you with food or ice cream for behaving well.

Now, this habit is not as difficult to change as emotional eating triggered by negative feelings. This sort of happy eating usually can be self-regulated. Understanding that your *health* is more important than *anything* related to unhealthy food is an excellent start to not faltering from our four-week plan.

I am not saying that you should not attend a celebration, just that you ask yourself if eating an entire loaf of bread with butter along with a big steak and all that comes with it is worth the way you will feel the next day. Think it through before you indulge impulsively. You most likely will not be the outcast in your company. In fact, you may be setting a good example. Saying that you are committed to a healthy lifestyle will quash any negative remarks.

Emotional eating can sabotage a healthy food plan and lead to feelings of guilt, regret, and self-hate.

The first step to controlling emotional eating is to distinguish between *real* hunger and emotional hunger. Anytime you get an impulse to eat, first ask yourself what you are *responding* to. Real hunger comes on gradually. You ultimately stop what you're doing because your stomach is speaking to you. You think about when you last ate a meal or a snack. You plan to eat if you haven't done so. If you are in a good place mentally and being conscientious about feeding your body with healthy meals, then you plan a nutritious meal or snack. Unless, of course, you haven't eaten for a long time. Then, of course, you will be ravenous and may go for an unhealthy choice. This is not emotional eating. This is downright real hunger!

If you are an emotional eater, it is likely that your body craves unhealthy food. Veggie soup just isn't going to sound tasty to you when you've been triggered by your emotional responses to eat. You are going to crave something sugary, like cookies; or creamy, like chocolate mousse; crunchy, like potato chips; or really fattening, like chicken parmesan with a side of pizza.

Why Are You an Emotional Eater?

There are several psychological reasons for emotional eating that I believe are best addressed in therapy with a licensed counselor. If you have had any sort of traumatic event in your life and you are medicating your feelings about it with food, then I suggest you look for a therapist who can help you address your specific needs. You might also consider joining a peer support group for overeaters.

Food is often used to fill a void. Identifying where this void is coming from is an essential step in stopping the reactional eating cycle. What is missing in your life that gives you an empty feeling that needs to be filled? Are you lonely? Have you suffered the loss of a person or a pet that had an important place in your life? Did you recently change your job?

Food also can be used as a distraction. Are you trying to get a project finished, but it seems overwhelming? Do you peruse your refrigeration or cabinets, randomly grazing, instead of buckling down and getting your work done?

Are you angry? You may be mad at a specific event or person. You may have overall anger with life in general. You may have underlying anger that you are unaware of, too. If you can relate to any of these reasons for anger, you may be eating to "stuff" your voice and your emotions. It takes bravery to voice your opinion when you're mad, especially when it may cause more conflict, so instead you eat to keep quiet and suppress the uncomfortable feelings.

Stress and anxiety are big reasons that your eating habits are currently out of control. Your hunger pangs may be a physical response to a rise in cortisol, a hormone that is elevated by stress. Your body thinks you need extra energy to fight stress and anxiety, so you head for the closest energy-producing type of food. Unfortunately, what your body thinks is right for you is not necessarily your best choice.

How Do You Cope?

To cope with emotional eating, I suggest that you begin by speaking with your physician. Check if you are on any medications that might be increasing your appetite. Perhaps you would benefit from medical treatment.

There are also many nonmedical ways to cope with the impulse to eat when you're not physically hungry. Some of these tips may help you.

- Keep a daily food diary. Writing down what you eat every day holds you more accountable.

- When you feel an intense craving comi
  yourself what you are really feeling. Ch
  yourself and determine if you are really hu..g.,
  when you last ate. Be sure to stay on a nutritionally
  healthy course throughout rough periods.
- Let the feelings come on. Don't try to stuff them down.
  Feelings are like the waves of the ocean. They ebb and
  flow. When I get an emotionally charged food craving,
  I take a moment to place my real feelings. I imagine
  myself sitting on the beach. I visualize a warm sunny
  day! The waves are coming in as if it were high tide.
  They are crashing at my feet. I feel what I'm feeling.
  Then I imagine the waves subsiding. I sit with this
  image for less than thirty seconds. Really, that is all it
  takes. The waves become calmer. The feelings drift.
  Find your own way of managing the ebb and flow of
  your emotions.
- Life is rarely a smooth sea. Its constant ups and downs
  are always going to be there. Know that these cravings
  are a temporary situation. Do a reality check.
- Find ways to manage stress. An immediate response
  is to head for the fast-food drive-through window or a
  candy aisle. Sometimes it helps to take a deep breath
  and count to ten. Breathe in as deeply as you can and
  then exhale all the air out from the top to the bottom
  of your lungs. Focusing on only your breath may be
  enough to get you grounded and reduce the stress to a

manageable proportion. Other, more permanent solutions might include taking a daily walk outside, joining a yoga or meditation class, or reading a book that has nothing to do with your own life.

The key to overall mental and physical well-being is to fill your life with positivity. The seven ways to balance your life that I shared with you in the Introduction can become the key elements of a healthy lifestyle. Sure, practicing the habits takes time and dedication, but it will have a significant reward for you in the future of your healthy lifestyle.

Getting Ready for Week Three

We spoke earlier about how excessively restrictive diets don't work. I would venture a guess that you would never have never made it this far with a previous plan if it was super limiting. Bad habits take time to break. But by now, any sugar addiction you had is already a dim memory. By the end of the second week, you will have given your taste buds the needed time to adjust and food will be tasting so much better. By this point, your exercise routine may be starting to provide you the oxygen that you have been missing for energy. Is your energy level rising?

Going into the third week of your new lifestyle is simple because by now you are starting to get the routine. The plan is making sense and you are feeling pretty darn good.

Starting This Monday

Keep going no matter what! Don't give up even if you haven't seen dramatic results yet. Think about how you are going to feel and look next beach season! In addition to planning healthy meals and doing your weekly shopping, be sure to write down on your schedule exactly when you will exercise. Remember that exercise is an appointment you make with yourself. Enter the days and times into your calendar that you intend to exercise this week.

WEEK TWO
EXERCISE & NUTRITION
JOURNAL

Starting This Monday

_____

_____

_____

_____

_____

_____

_____

_____

_____

_____

_____

_____

_____

_____

_____

_____

_____

_____

_____

_____

_____

WEEK THREE

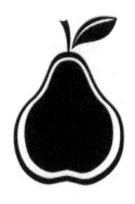

THE SKINNY ON FATS

"Live one day at a time."[1]
Alcoholics Anonymous

Week Three is about getting rid of fats that are bad for you. When focusing on eliminating unhealthy fats from your diet, a good place to start is by eliminating trans-fats.

Since you are on Week Three, you may have already removed almost all, if not all, trans-fats from your diet over the past two weeks. If so, this step is going to be easy.

Here is the skinny on bad fats, starting with the worst. *Trans-unsaturated fatty acids* (aka *trans-fats*) are an unhealthy substance, also known as *trans-fatty acids* or *partially hydrogenated oil. Hydrogenation* is a chemical process that solidifies liquid oils. This is done to increase the shelf life, flavor, and stability of oils and the processed foods that contain them. Trans-fat begins as a normal fat molecule and then becomes deformed through processing. This oil is ideal for frying in fast-food restaurants as it can be repeatedly heated to extreme temperatures without breaking down. It is a chemical process that is good for food manufacturing, but really bad for your health. In recent years, it has been banned in some locales because it is terrible for us.

Trans-fats wreak havoc on the body's ability to regulate cholesterol. In the list of fats from good to bad, trans-fats are considered the worst. This type of fat elevates cholesterol, which increases your risk of arterial heart disease and stroke.[2] Studies have shown that this fat may also be responsible for the growth of cancer cells. According to the FDA, those who consume above six and a half grams of trans-fat per day raise their risk for colon polyps by 86 percent.[3]

That statistic is mind-blowing to me.

Another study of 25,000 women showed that those who ate trans-fat were twice as likely to develop breast cancer.[4] Because of multiple findings like these, the FDA has ruled that trans-fats are no longer generally recognized as safe for use in food.[5]

Foods you would find in a typical grocery store that still contain trans-fats include vegetable shortening and some margarine, crackers, cookies, cake mixes, and snack foods. Trans-fats are also found in abundance in fried foods.

Vegetable oil is also not the best option. I do not use any type of vegetable oil when I cook. Like the chemical process of making white flour, vegetable oils have their own highly processed manufacturing. They may be refined, bleached, or deodorized and may contain any number of different oils, among them canola (rapeseed) oil, corn oil, sunflower oil, cottonseed oil, and soy oil. I prefer to know that what I ingest has high nutritional value, is not overly processed, and has clear ingredients listed on the label so I can avoid these oils.

Let's conclude that trans-fats are humanmade by industrial processing, and definitely not good for you.

Fats That Are Healthy to Eat

The following list will help you figure out what foods to eat to help lower your fat intake.

Good (healthy) fats to consume come from ingredients that include avocados, olives, flaxseeds, sesame seeds, sunflower seeds, pumpkin seeds, almonds, walnuts, cashews—and many other nuts—and fish like tuna, salmon, and sardines.

Every oil is unique in its nature. My favorite to cook with is extra-virgin olive oil. It is full of nutrients and mildly processed. Be aware, however, that it does have a low smoke point, which means it cannot be heated to high temperatures. Once the oil is overheated beyond its smoke point, the flavor is compromised, and it can become unhealthy.

Avocado oil is a good choice for a higher smoke point oil. It's a good choice for recipes that require a higher heat, such as stir fry. Another great choice for high-heat cooking is sesame oil. I love the taste of stir fry when I use sesame oil, and I bet you will too.

I love grass-fed butter, and I do cook with it. However, if I'm putting on a few extra pounds, butter (and cheese) are the first to go—even the grass-fed variety. Be moderate in your consumption of dairy. A small number of dairy products can log in a lot of calories.

Low-fat cheese is a reasonable substitute in cooking as it has the same nutritional value as full-fat cheeses. The catch is you may find the taste bland; if you're not careful, you could end up consuming more while chasing flavor.

Whenever possible, buy grass-fed and organic dairy and meat. Remember my conversation with you regarding poisons used in crop fields. These crops are used to feed and graze animals, so anything they eat, you also eat.

Tips to Replace "Bad" Fats

During Week Three, begin swapping in healthy fats for unhealthy fats. For example:

- Dress your baked potato with low-fat plain yogurt instead of butter and sour cream.
- At breakfast, enjoy turkey or chicken sausage instead of pork sausage.
- Use mustard instead of mayo.

- Bake sliced sweet potato or white potato coated with a small quantity of extra-virgin olive oil instead of deep-frying it in oil.

When eating out, skip the fried foods, biscuits, and bacon. Skip anything that is typically presented doused in cream sauce, brown sauce, or butter sauce. These entrees are drowned in fat and very often sugar.

Another way of cutting fats from your diet is to eat less red meat. When you do choose red meat, choose lean cuts. Eat more fish, chicken, and lean pork. Remove the skin from the chicken and eat only the white meat. The same goes for turkey.

Choose low-fat or fat-free milk, yogurt, cheese, and other dairy products. And stick to the main philosophy of eating "clean," whole foods. If you can't identify the ingredients in something, then don't eat it!

Add Healthy Movement to Your New Lifestyle

As you progress into your new lifestyle of movement, healthy eating, and a more toxin-free environment, it may be time to look at some other methods of implementing healthy ways of getting out of your old habits and filling your world with new positive experiences. This is also a learning process. You won't know until you try something new whether you like it or not. Since you are already doing some resistance exercises with your water jugs, or maybe you have joined a gym, I suggest you try tai chi or yoga. You don't have to be flexible, thin, or have peace and love symbols hanging from your neck to delve into this sort of practice. You do have to be willing to try something new and understand that the word *practice* is the key to the whole thing. Being able to balance on one leg doesn't come overnight to most of us, and it doesn't really matter at all how fast you progress. These sort of practices take us on a personal journey to expand our capabilities a little a time.

Be sure to consult a medical doctor before you begin your practice. If you are pregnant, my suggestion is to steer towards a tai chi or yoga class specifically designed for your condition. Be sure to tell your instructor if you are pregnant or have any other conditions that need modifications.

I do not have much personal experience with tai chi, so I will talk a little about yoga. There are many reasons that yoga is beneficial.

All yoga poses can be modified to suit your individual needs. Initially you may discover your range of motion is extremely limited. Don't be hard on yourself. Flexibility takes time. As does learning the practice of calming your nervous system and your mind, all of the things that make yoga a "practice." Do what you can today, and then tomorrow, or the day after that, you may be able to do a little more.

Yoga Increases Lung Capacity

Take a moment to see how deeply you can breathe. Many of us are not taking the time to deepen our breath, drop our shoulders from up by our ears, and give our lungs the full attention they deserve. We need oxygen in our bodies to function. Sitting in **Easy pose** (see below) will help you get in the habit of breathing deeply. The Sanskrit name for this pose is *Sukhasana*.

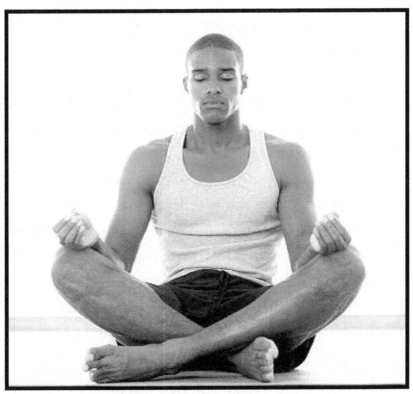

Easy pose (*Sukhasana*). Photo © GlobalStock via iStock
by Getty Images.

Here are the steps to do Easy pose.

1. Fold a blanket and place it underneath your bottom so that you are sitting with your hips slightly above your knees. Sit on the edge of the blanket.
2. Bring your legs straight out in front of you.
3. Fold your shins in a cross-legged position.
4. Press the outside of both soles of your feet firmly down.
5. Take a deep breath and sit up straight, shoulders back and relaxed. Do not arch your back.
6. Be sure you are sitting evenly on your buttocks.
7. Move your tailbone towards the floor.
8. Lay your hands gently on top of each other, palms facing up, or rest them gently on your knees, palms facing down.
9. Stay in Easy pose for as long as you are comfortable. You can stay in this pose for as long as you wish but be sure to uncross your legs and then cross with the opposite shin in front. Give equal time to both sides.
10. To come out of the pose, ease yourself forward onto your hands and knees, and then place one leg forward with a bent knee and with the strength of your front leg, hands on thigh, stand up.

Modification: Sit in a chair with your feet grounded into the floor.

Yoga Can Be Meditative

Consider how many thoughts race through your mind at any given moment. This is exhausting for your brain. If your brain is tired, your entire well-being is compromised. Settling peacefully into a yoga position such **Child's pose** (see below) while focusing only on your breath will ease your mind and bring calm to your body. As thoughts come in, gently let them go as if they are clouds drifting through your mind. Continue to bring your awareness back to your breath. The Sanskrit name for this pose is *Balasana*.

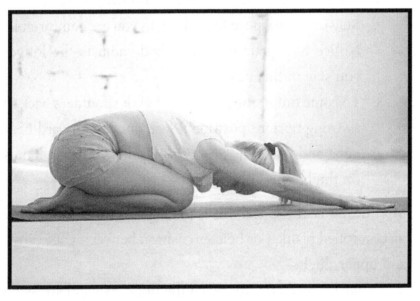

Child's pose (*Balasana*). Photo © fizkes via iStock by Getty Images.

Here are the steps to do Child's pose.

1. Kneel on the floor with your knees wide and toes touching.
2. Sit your butt on your heels.
3. Keeping your back straight, lower your torso forward to rest on or between your thighs with your head on a mat in front of you.
4. Try to continue to keep your butt on your heels.
5. Extend your arms out in front of you, palms down, or keep them at your side, near your heels.
6. Continue breathing with deep, flowing breaths.
7. Stay in Child's pose for as long as you are comfortable. Notice how your mind and body adjusts the longer you stay in this position.
8. To come out of the pose, kneel with shoulders back in a strong upright position. Place one leg forward bent knee and with the strength of your front leg, hands on thigh, stand up.

Modifications: If you feel this is putting stress on your knees, place a rolled blanket or bolster cushion between your calves and upper thighs.

If your forehead cannot reach the floor, to avoid stress on your neck, place a rolled blanket or bolster under your forehead.

Yoga Helps Us Become More Flexible

You don't need to be flexible to start a yoga practice. And you never need to be as flexible as a ballet dancer. However, it *is* important for you to be flexible so you can move freely and enjoy your activities. Flexibility is important for overall muscle and joint health. Joints must be able to work in a full range of motion to help prevent injuries and overall stiffness in the body. Try **Downward-facing Dog pose** (see below) for a total stretch of the backside of your body from heels to head! The Sanskrit name for this pose is *Adho Mukha Svanasana.*

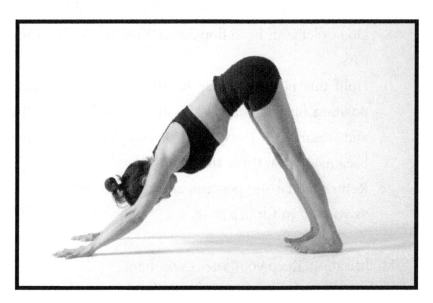

Downward-facing Dog pose (*Adho Mukha Svanasana*).
Photo: © solidcolours via iStock by Getty Images.

Here are the steps to do Downward-facing Dog pose.

1. Begin on your hands and knees. (Your wrists should be directly under your shoulders).
2. Tuck your toes.
3. Press strongly into your knuckles and palms as you lift your hips towards the ceiling.
4. Gently straighten your legs, without locking your knees. You are aiming to be in an upside-down V.
5. Continue raising your hips and pressing them back at the same time.
6. Descend your heels towards to ground. But don't be concerned if your heels don't entirely reach the floor.
7. Your backside from head to tailbone should be flat.
8. Do not let your head flop down. Keep it between your ears.
9. Hold this pose for three breaths, return to starting position on your hands and knees for three breaths and return to Downward Facing Dog for three breaths. Repeat three times.
10. Return to starting position and come to exit the pose as you did in Child's pose.

Modification: Keep your knees very bent.

Yoga Enhances the Mind-Body Connection

Because yoga principles enhance the connection between mind and body, yoga can be empowering. My favorite pose is **Warrior One pose** (see next page) with the arms raised to the sky and touching, almost like a prayer, or like your body has become an arrow that's pointing toward the sun. This pose requires stability, strength, and concentration. Its Sanskrit name is *Virabhadrasana*. Try Warrior One and feel how mentally and physically strong this pose can make you feel.

Here are the steps to do Warrior One pose.

1. Begin standing with feet a little more than hip-width apart.
2. Step one leg backwards and bend your front leg into a lunge. Your knee should be in line with your ankle, not in front of it. Lengthen your stance if necessary.
3. Turn out your back foot 90 degrees.
4. Turn in your front foot slightly 45 degrees.
5. Keep both of your hips squared forward.
6. Reach up powerfully through your arms and touch your hands palm to palm.
7. Gaze upwards beyond your hands.

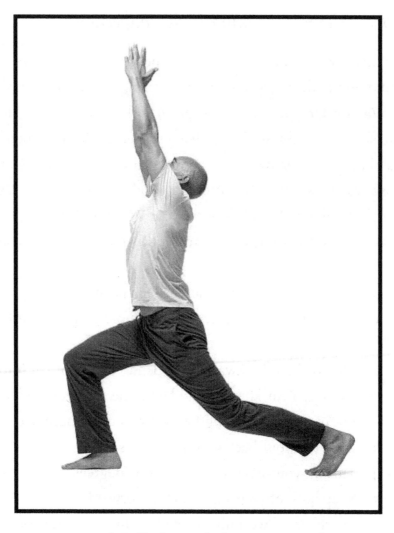

Warrior One (*Virabhadrasana*). Photo © Neustockimages
via iStock by Getty Images.

8. Stay in Warrior for a minute or more and notice your body adjusting to the power of the pose.To exit the pose, you may need to wiggle your feet together and stand tall. Take a deep breath.

9. Repeat the entire sequence with the other leg.

Modifications: To increase your stability, you may separate your legs, so they are wider apart.

You may keep your arms wide at the top (rather than touching palms), gazing upward between them, or place your hands on your hips and gaze forward.

Yoga Improves Posture

Typically, we sit. We drive. We schlump. We carry stuff and get in the habit of leaning to one side or the other. We are injured. Among all of the other poses that also work on body alignment **Mountain pose** (see next page) is the one to practice for standing up straight. Mastering this pose is a practice in itself. At its essence, Mountain Pose is active standing. It has many benefits. The Sanskrit name for this pose is *Tadasana*.

Here are the steps to do Mountain pose.

1. Stand tall with your big toes together and your heels slightly apart. Hands are at your sides, palms slightly facing away from you.

2. Elevate your heels by coming up on the balls of your feet.

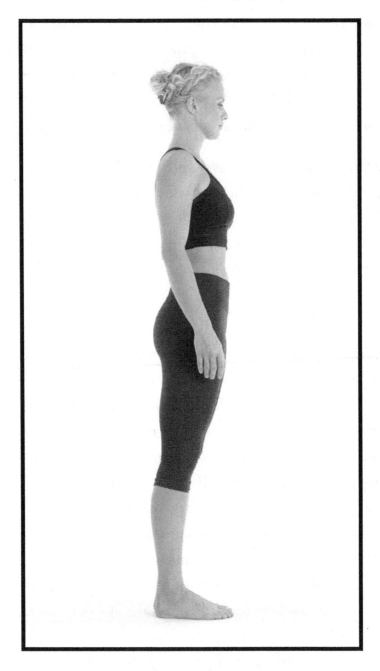

Mountain pose (*Tadasana*). Photo © In Pictures via iStock by Getty Images.

3. Lower your heels while keeping your big toes together.

4. Stand firmly and equally on both the balls of your feet and your heels. Raise your toes slightly while you press your pinky toes and big toes firmly down.

5. Keep your thighs engaged and tuck your tailbone.

6. Elongate your torso without changing your tailbone.

7. Raise your sternum (breastbone) upward without arching your back.

8. Widen your collarbones.

9. Relax your shoulders away from your ears.

10. Imagine a magnet moving your crown (the top of your head) upward while planting your feet firmly down.

11. Do not raise your chin—keep it level.

12. Keep your gaze forward.

13. Breathe deeply without changing your structure.

14. Stay in Mountain Pose for as long as it takes you to make all the minor adjustments needed for beautiful alignment.

Modifications: For help with balance, stand with your feet apart or close to a chair.

You can try this pose first with your heels, lower back, shoulder blades, and the back of your head against a wall.

Yoga Improves Balance

Balance is important, especially as we age. As we get older, the receptors in our brains become, well, old. They don't work quite as effectively. The tendency to lose equilibrium can put us in dangerous situations. Practicing balancing poses can help delay this process. We can teach our minds and bodies to find our center of gravity and be aware of our strength and alignment.

Learning how to root your feet and ground downward not only will help your balance, it also will help you when you're feeling flighty or out of control. **Tree pose** (see next page), which is known as *Vrksasana* in Sanskrit, is the one to try.

Here are the steps to do Tree pose.

1. Start in Mountain pose (see page 80).
2. Bring your hands to your hips.
3. Without changing your hips, which are facing forward, shift your weight to one leg. Pause for a moment.
4. Raise your knee opposite the standing leg outward and rest the moving foot either above or below the knee of your standing leg.
5. Bring your hands forward in front of you, palms and fingers together in prayer position in front of your chest. You have the choice to raise them over your head.
6. Root your standing foot into the ground.

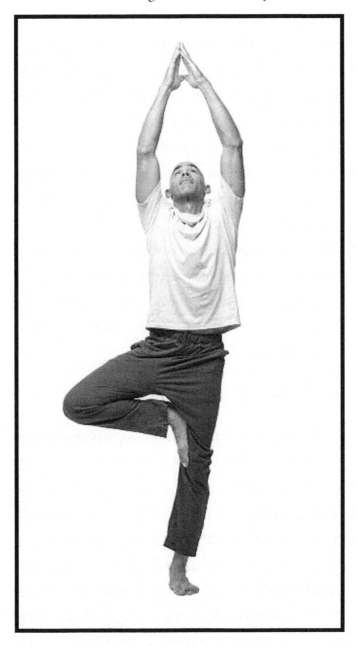

Tree pose (*Vrksasana*). Photo © Neustockimages
via iStock by Getty Images.

7. Imagine yourself as a tree. Gaze in front of you to one spot. Keep your core muscles engaged.

8. Stay in Tree pose for as long as you can keep your balance. Aim to take five to ten breaths, then return to your starting position.

9. Repeat the sequence on the other side.

10. Notice the difference on each side. You may find that your balance is better on one side. That is completely normal.

Modifications: Stand next to a chair or the wall in case you feel wobbly and may need support.

Instead of bringing your foot above or below your knee, you may rest it on the ground with your heel against your ankle.

Yoga Helps Us Reduce Anxiety and Stress

One of the many principles behind yoga philosophy is that your mind and body are one. As a mind-body practice, yoga brings awareness to all aspects of the body. Among other benefits, yoga helps to develop self-awareness and emotional control through breathing, learning to focus the mind, and releasing emotional blocks. **Half Standing Forward Bend pose** (see page 94) is an excellent pose to reduce stress. Supported forward bend is a nice way to give yourself a moment to unwind and reset your thoughts. Whenever a teacher friend of mine goes into this pose using her desk, her students know that they better behave. The Sanskrit name for this pose is *Uttanasana.*

Here are the steps to do Half Standing Forward Bend pose. You will need a chair, the back of a couch, a table, or a desk to do it.

1. Begin standing with your feet hip-width apart.
2. Bend your knees slightly.
3. Stand upright and tall.
4. Pressing your heels down into the floor, fold forward, hinging at your hips. Press your hips behind you.
5. Keep your chest upright and shoulders back.
6. Place your hands on your thighs or shins. Your position will resemble a tabletop. Be aware of not overarching your lower back.
7. Keep your head neutral—don't look up or drop your chin down low.
8. Stay in this position for as long as you wish. Notice how the longer you stay the more restored your energy becomes.
9. To return to starting position, keep your knees soft, place your hands on your waist and gently with the strength of your upper body stand tall.

Modifications: Fold your arms on the back of a chair or on a table. Rest your forehead on your folded arms.

If you are very flexible, you may continue all the way to the floor with your hands. Keep your knees soft.

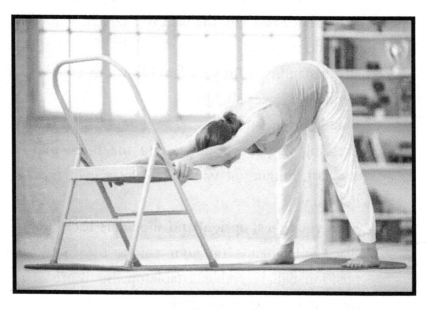

Modified Half Standing Forward Bend pose (*Uttanasana*), done using a chair for support. Photo © valentinrussanov via iStock by Getty Images.

Yoga Improves the Circulatory System

Movement of any sort can improve circulation. Circulation supplies oxygen, blood, and nutrients to the vital organs. The way that yoga combines breathing with specific movements is super beneficial. **Legs Up the Wall pose** (see page 96) is relaxing and rejuvenating, especially if you have been either sitting for a long time or on your feet all day. In this pose, you are reversing your body, and it gives you an opportunity to rest at a deep level. The Sanskrit name for this pose is *Viparita Karani.*

Here are the steps to do Legs Up the Wall pose. The trick to entering this pose successfully is to get your buttocks as close to the wall as possible before you lay down.

1. Sit facing to one side of the wall with one hip against the wall.
2. Gradually lower your body while working your legs up the wall. You will end up in an L form on your back.
3. Relax your lower back and let your thighs completely release.
4. Let your toes point down towards you.
5. Stay as long in the pose as long as you like.
6. To exit this pose, wiggle away from the wall. Bend your knees towards your chest and roll to either side. Rest for a moment in fetal position. Come on to all fours, and then to a kneeling position. Bend one leg forward and with the strength of your hands on your forward thigh stand tall. Give yourself a minute to adjust from being upside down.

Modification: If lying flat puts strain on your lower back, then place a rolled up blanket under your hips.

It is not possible to get your legs all the way up the wall, then it's OK to keep your buttocks slightly away from the wall. You may also rest your bent legs on a chair seat.

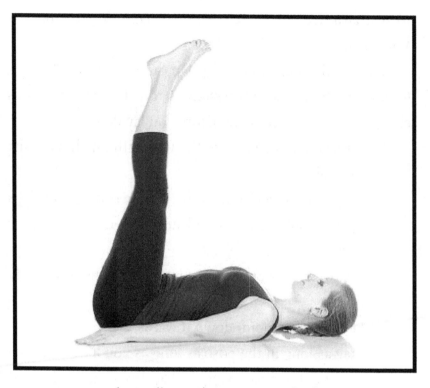

Legs Up the Wall pose (*Viparita Karani*). Photo ©
byheaven via iStock by Getty Images.

Getting Ready for Week Four

It is not easy to do what you have done in these last three
weeks. In the overall scheme of your life, three weeks is just
a blip in time. But I know that this journey, when you are in
it feels long. Keep in mind that it is easier to get through this
major mind-blowing life change now than to look back later
on if you haven't yet and wish you had done it sooner. Don't
wait for some profound moment that you hope will arrive to
give you the strength and courage and discipline to change

the inevitable. And please don't wait until you are ill. Do it now so that you can look back with pride. You have the ability to move to the future without regrets.

WEEK THREE
EXERCISE & NUTRITION
JOURNAL

Starting This Monday

WEEK FOUR

LIVING A HEALTHY LIFE IS MEDICINE

Food is medicine.

You are probably beginning to see how the mind and body synergistically work together. Hopefully, you are connecting your outer self to your inner world through better habits and choices. By now, you may be seeing changes in your mental acuity as well as in your strength and endurance. You may be "getting it"! You may be embracing the notion that your body truly is a temple. Can you keep up the momentum for another week?

Take Responsibility and Talk to Your Doctor about Options

If you are a person who is chronically ill and medicates with pharmaceuticals, and yet eats an unhealthy diet and does little or no exercise, then you have not grasped the concept of holistic living yet. Living a healthy life *is* medicine. Nutrient-dense food *is* medicine. Exercise *is* medicine. There are many options available to us besides pharmacology. Speak to your doctor about what lifestyle modifications you should make to reduce your reliance on drugs.

If you truly care about your outcome in life, then be your own advocate by taking responsibility and considering your options. Research your ailments and ask questions before you commit to taking pills or having surgery. Find a medical practitioner who is willing to listen to your questions and suggest alternatives to pharmaceuticals. Ask yourself if you are living a holistic life. Combined with modern medicine it is ultimately up to you to come up with solutions.

Caution: Never stop taking prescription medication abruptly without consulting your personal physician or other health care provider.

Grocery Shopping Can Be a Life-Promoting Activity

It is imperative to embrace the mindset that shopping for groceries can be a potentially life-changing event. This is a weekly experience that takes practice to do well! Find ways to make it fun and easy for yourself to shop for the healthy ingredients you need to stay on plan. If you have a family (spouse or partner and/or kids), engage them, and ask each of them to come up with a healthy recipe that you all can enjoy together.

Add those ingredients to your food list.

Choose at least one new recipe from the Recipes Ideas chapter that follows this one and add its ingredients to your shopping list too.

To save time, keep Your Basic Shopping List available and add to it as you go (see pages 20–21). One of the ways to make keeping a comprehensive food list easier is to keep track of the products that you prefer—the ones that have already passed your assessment. For example, if you're looking for a healthy chicken broth, and you spend ten minutes sorting through all the ones that have additives (which you don't consume any more) and you finally find one that has ingredients you approve of, then write that brand name down. That way you can avoid needing to do the same assessment twice.

Did you find sugar-free ketchup? Log the brand name.

Did you find a bread bakery that uses only ingredients on your checklist and none of the contraindicated ingredients? Frequent that bakery!

The idea of shopping for items on sale is no longer on your radar. The idea is to shop for what is on your list and to hope that the item is on sale. Your overall wellbeing—your being—is much more important than a few dollars. You will be less sick and need to take less time off work if you consume real, wholesome food. We can't put a price on health.

Time for a Progress Evaluation: How Well Is This Plan Working for You?

You have been on course now for three weeks. It is time to reevaluate what you have done. This is a good time to think about a reward. Maybe you have your eye on a new outfit, a vacation, a massage, a new pair of sneakers, or even a food that you are really missing. Look back over these last few weeks and take note of how you feel now compared to when you started. It took determination to get here, but you did it!

Before beginning, you committed to being *well* and cleaned out your home of all foods that are not on the plan.

During Week One, you detoxed yourself from sugar, *and* you started an exercise plan.

During Week Two, you rid yourself of white flour.

During Week Three, you said good-bye to high-fat meats and dairy foods and other unhealthy fats.

You have been on a mission to have overall health and wellness. Maybe you wanted to lose weight. You desired energy and vibrancy. Now, you are looking at your body as a place of worship, and you are taking care of yourself so you can be a better version of yourself.

How's your weight?

How's your energy?

What, if anything, has changed during the past three weeks?

Maybe It's Time to Do More?

If you have followed the guidelines presented to you within the past three weeks, and you aren't where you want to be yet, then it's time now, in the fourth week, to look at some additional factors that could be stopping you from getting healthy.

Be sure that there are no underlying medical issues, such as thyroid, diabetes, and hormonal or metabolic ailments. If all is well medically and you aren't seeing a change on the scale, then the reason is usually too much food, not enough exercise or both.

Being completely honest with yourself, is there any habit you haven't broken yet? Are you 100 percent free of all added sugar, white flour products, and fried foods? If so, and you haven't given up alcohol yet, now is the time to do so.

The Trouble of Alcohol and Weight Loss

Alcohol is high in calories, so pay attention to the caloric content of the cocktails you are consuming. If you're drinking alcohol mixed with fruit juices, there will be even more calories in your beverages than if you drink alcohol neat or mixed with seltzer water.

Remember, the idea when trying to lose weight and be overall healthier is to consume nutrient-rich foods and beverages while ingesting the minimum amount of calories. Careful planning of your calorie consumption is the key to losing weight and keeping it off, as well as helping to assure a healthy, illness-free life. A balanced diet will curb hunger and provide the necessary nutrients for health and wellness.

When trying to live "clean," it is a simple decision to forego alcohol. Alcohol is not a necessary element of a healthy diet. Instead, it can provide a lot of calories and negatively impact many aspects of your health for other reasons. It makes you tipsy (or drunk) because it's essentially poisoning your liver.

If you choose to drink, you will need to limit the quantity and type of alcohol you consume. Sugary mixed drinks and sugary premade mixers are an absolute NO. But you have already removed refined sugar, so it is time to count the calories from alcohol to fit within your daily goal.

Have you ever noticed that anytime you drink alcohol, you feel hungrier or end up eating more than usual? That's because alcohol impairs your judgment, lowers your willpower, and stimulates your desire for food. Because it can increase feelings of hunger, especially, this combination is setting you up for failure if you are trying to follow this program to the letter.

In addition, there are a vast number of nutrients that become depleted in your body with excess alcohol consumption. Here are some of them[2]:

- **Folate:** Folate is part of the B vitamin family. It helps the body to produce and maintain red blood cells, preventing anemia. It is a support to the nervous system and helps produce DNA. Alcohol interferes with dietary folate intake and absorption.

- **Vitamin B12:** The body uses Vitamin B12 to make protein and to maintain healthy nerves and red blood cells. According to MedicineNet, "Studies have shown that both moderate and heavy alcohol consumption will affect vitamin B12 levels."[3]

- **Vitamin A:** Vitamin A is needed for healthy eyesight, immunity, the growth of bones, and reproduction, as well as cell division and differentiation. It is fat soluble and toxic in high doses—and alcohol apparently increases its toxicity!

- **Calcium:** Without sufficient calcium, your bones would get brittle and break easily, a debilitating condition known as osteoporosis. In addition to building bones with it, your body uses calcium for muscle contraction and expansion, to keep blood vessels healthy, to secrete hormones and enzymes, and for communication through the nervous system. Alcohol consumption can cause a loss of calcium.

Many vitamin and mineral deficiencies occur when the "empty" (no-value) calories in alcohol replace those from other ingredients in a balanced diet. It also can cause damage to your liver and other organs, may lead to a high triglyceride profile and high or low blood sugar, and contribute to stomach ulcers.

If your diet and health plan have room (calorically speaking) for you to indulge in a few drinks, then, yes, there may be occasional benefits to drinking in moderation. We have all heard that red wine is beneficial for the heart, that tequila stimulates the metabolism, and that a nice bourbon warms the soul. But proceed according to your personal guidelines, which you are setting up now for a healthier future.

Exercise: No One Is Looking at You

It's important that you take a fresh look at your exercise program this week. Are you pushing the twenty-minute protocol every day? If you haven't lost weight yet, and want to, you may want to reserve additional time for your exercise regimen. At least two or three days a week, burn more calories by adding ten to twenty minutes of exercise to each session.

The other option is to lower your calorie intake.

Or you can do both—get more exercise and consume fewer calories!

There are numerous reasons why people don't exercise. I have heard too many to list, but some of the top conversations I have had in my career are:

Client: "I worked all day, so I don't need to go to the gym."
Me: "Really? Did you do some weight training and cardio at work while at your desk?"

Client: "I work construction, so I get plenty of exercise."
Me: "Oh, wow! Yes, that's a hard job, what do you do?"
Client: "I sit in the cab and work the bucket loader."

Client: "My kids keep me busy, so I have no time."
Me: "Do you homeschool them? Or are they in school for most of the day?"

Client: "I am injured, I think I hurt my shoulder."
Me: "Do you have other body parts available to work out?"

"I don't like to sweat. . . ."
"I can't get up early. . . ."
"I want to go home after work. . . ."

I've heard every excuse you could imagine. My personal favorite is:

Client: "I need to lose weight before I go to the gym."
Me: "*What?* No one is looking at you."

The point is that exercise is a commitment and a schedule you make with yourself. Even though you might be busy at work or working a physical job, this doesn't mean that you have a balanced physical program in place. If you haul lumber all day, your back may be strong, but your core may be weak. If you stand all day, your legs may be strong, but the rest of your body may be weak. If you are sitting at a desk, you could end up with rounded shoulders and many other muscular, skeletal, and cardiovascular problems unless you stretch and exercise.

A healthy exercise program involves cardiovascular activity to bring oxygen to your bloodstream, heart, and lungs; weight training for skeletal strength, alignment, and bone density; and stretching for body alignment and flexibility.

Discovering the Individual Needs of Your Body

In addition to the exercise component, be sure that you are accurate when measuring your food portions. It may help to get a food scale. There's no excuse not to, because many scales are inexpensive. Using a scale at first is helpful because it will help train your eye for the future so that when you are trying to add up your calories you will be accurate about your intake.

I won't recommend a specific amount of calories for you. There are many factors in determining how many calories you need to cut back to lose weight. These factors include how much exercise you are getting every day and your age. The amount to cut back also depends on how much weight you need to lose and how much muscle mass you carry. Muscle burns more calories than fat, so if you have good muscle tone, you may need to eat more calories per day than a less muscular person.

If you start losing weight too quickly, you may need to add calories. If you're losing too slowly, you may need to decrease calories. I want you to get to know your body and learn what it needs well enough that you do not have to count calories or weigh your food.

By the end of Week Four, you will have spent a whole month getting to know yourself better, and to understand what types of emotional triggers cause you to want to eat beyond what you need to survive and fuel your body. You will get to know yourself even better as time goes on and proper nutrition and exercise become a bigger part of your life.

What It Takes to Stay the Course

As I mentioned earlier, living the healthy life you envisioned takes dedication. It's not just about nutritious food that you are now eating; it's about replacing negative behaviors with positive experiences. The more you fill up your life with positive experiences, the less time you have for emotional eating and toxic behavior. Combining inner health and outward health—meaning, focusing on creating health of mind as well as health of body—will help you achieve balance and make good choices every day.

Very often, jobs, kids, and life in general take over your need to care for yourself. Sometimes this has been going on so long that you don't remember how to have fun. Perhaps your hobbies have been put on a back shelf, or you feel like you don't have a moment to reflect. Maybe when you were growing up, you never learned about balance and nutrition.

"Whatever you hold in your mind on a consistent basis is exactly what you will experience in your life."[3]
—Tony Robbins

Replace every negative behavior and thought you have with more positive ones. Take on your poor habits one at a time and replace them with good habits. Before you know it, your life will be full and balanced. You will eventually get to a point where you can control your eating habits so well that having dessert after dinner or eating a slice of pizza won't throw you off course and spiral you into months of eating poorly and sabotaging your body. Attaining good health is a thinking-and-doing process.

At first, swapping positive for negative behaviors might not come naturally, but time and practice will make you a pro at it, and you will not only admire yourself but be a good role model for those around you. If you have children, you can teach them by example how to balance their lives with good nutrition, exercise, surrounding themselves with positive people, and making overall good choices. Besides saving yourself from illness and death, you are saving them as well by demonstrating what to do. You are learning and teaching that even though you don't feel like it, you are going to do it anyway. This means not only in what you eat and how much you exercise but in your lifestyle itself.

I hope that during the last three weeks, besides the nutritional changes you made, you have been able to implement some of the seven components of a balanced and fulfilling life. As you take on the advice in Week Four, it moves you into the future.

The future is up to you—so stay the course.

Always remember that you are the captain of your ship.

WEEK FOUR
EXERCISE & NUTRITION
JOURNAL

Starting This Monday

--

RECIPE IDEAS

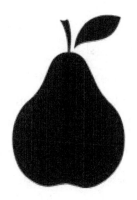

I have tried to make these recipes as simple as possible while trying to be creative at the same time. You can make any of these without fancy equipment. For each recipe, I have indicated a number of servings. This is intended to give you a rough idea of how many people the recipe will be able to serve. It is not based on government guidelines, but on my own family's appetite. If you have hungry teenagers in your household and the recipe calls for one chicken breast to serve per person, you can adjust your ingredients accordingly to accommodate the precise needs of your family of two or four or six wildly or mildly hungry people, as the case may be.

If you were to ask me what equipment to purchase besides basic pots and pans, I would suggest an Instant Pot or another brand of pressure cooker and a Ninja® or other high-speed blender. The Instant Pot cuts cooking time down usually by more than half, and the meats turn out as tender as could possibly be, while the veggies remain firm. You can cook just about anything in this one piece of kitchenware, including hard-boiled eggs!

My Ninja® blender was given to me by a client as a gift. I was going to continue to struggle along with my old blender. I am beyond grateful! I use the Ninja® nearly daily to make smoothies. It blends the ice and frozen fruits and veggies so much better than a blender! I also use it to make juices, hummus, and other dips, and I blend soups with it. It's got good bang for the buck.

Soups are so easy to make and easily frozen. Salads don't have to be boring with just lettuce and tomatoes. You can really do up a fancy salad by using lots of colors. Yellow, red, and green Bell peppers, orange carrots, red tomato, purple cabbage, light green cucumbers, different-colored beans—for example, garbanzos (beige), kidney (dark red), or black—and sliced hard-boiled eggs (yellow and white). I always make my own salad dressing.

I keep my kitchen super simple. I cook with just the basics. The Basic Shopping List I shared with you in the chapter on Preparation is my personal day-to-day go-to shopping list. Because you are acclimating to a new and healthier way of living, I suggest simplicity for now—deliberately not getting complicated. As you learn how to cook healthfully, you will be able to expand your repertoire and become more creative.

Starting This Monday

When I am invited to someone's home and have been asked to bring something, I usually will bring a large vegetable platter and hummus. This way, even if there are no healthy food options presented to me, I am never stuck with nothing to eat. If I have the time, I will bring something even more creative that is nonetheless healthy.

CLASSIC HUMMUS

Makes 4–6 servings

Hummus is versatile. It can take on many fun flavors, depending upon your ingredients. It is so easy to prepare, in fact, that you can make a few different flavors and present these in small bowls served with sliced veggies. You can use a food processor, blender, potato masher, mortar stone and pestle, or smoothie maker to make this dish.

INGREDIENTS

15-1/2 oz. can garbanzo beans (drained and rinsed)
3 T fresh-squeezed lemon juice
1 garlic clove
1/2 cup tahini (or creamy sugar-free peanut butter)
1/4 tsp salt
1/4 tsp fresh ground pepper
1/4 tsp cumin
3-1/2 T olive oil
3-1/2 T cold water

Note: Shake the tahini well before measuring, as the oil tends to separate.

INSTRUCTIONS

1. Add all of the above ingredients together. Blend until almost smooth.
2. Empty into a bowl and drizzle a little olive oil on top.
3. Serve at room temperature with vegetables.

VARIATIONS

You can add any ingredients to hummus to make it your own. Here are my three favorites.

Option 1. Kalamata Olive Hummus. Include 1/2 cup pitted and drained kalamata olives to the other ingredients. Blend everything together. Pour into a serving bowl. Chop up a few olives and sprinkle the pieces on top.

Option 2. Roasted Red Pepper Hummus. Add 3/4 cup roasted red peppers (drained) to the other ingredients. Replace the cumin with 1/4 tsp smoked paprika powder. Blend everything together. Pour into a serving bowl. Chop a few roasted peppers and sprinkle the pieces on top.

Option 3. Lemon and Sage Hummus. Replace the cold water with 3-1/2 T fresh lemon juice. (The total lemon juice thus becomes 6-1/2 T). Add 1/2 tsp sage powder. Blend well. Pour in a serving dish.

WHITE BEAN AND SPINACH DIP

Makes 4 servings

You can use a food processor, blender, potato masher, mortar stone and pestle, or smoothie maker to prepare this dish.

INGREDIENTS

15-1/2 oz. can of cannellini beans (drained and rinsed)
3 T fresh-squeezed lemon juice
2 large cloves garlic chopped
2 compacted cups fresh baby spinach
3-1/2 T olive oil, divided
2 T. cold water
1 tsp ground sage or T fresh chopped sage
1/4 tsp salt
1/4 tsp ground black pepper

INSTRUCTIONS

1. Chop the garlic and sauté in 1 T olive oil (reserve the rest of the oil). When it is light brown, remove the garlic from the oil and set it aside to cool.
2. Sauté the spinach in 2 T olive oil. When the leaves are wilted (in 20–30 seconds) remove and cool. Drain as

much liquid from the spinach as you can. Blot with a paper towel. Set aside.

3. Blend until almost smooth the beans, garlic, lemon juice, 2 T olive oil, cold water, sage, salt, and pepper.
4. Chop the spinach removing any larger stems. Stir by hand into the bean mixture.
5. Drizzle the remaining 1/2 T. of olive oil on top.
6. Serve chilled or at room temperature with veggies.

OLD BAY® SEASONED DEVILED EGGS

Makes 6 servings

Everybody loves deviled eggs. The Old Bay® Seasoning kicks them up a notch.

INGREDIENTS

6 hard-boiled eggs
4 T low-fat sour cream or thick nonfat Greek- or Scandinavian-style plain yogurt
1/2 tsp yellow mustard
1 tsp Old Bay® Seasoning
Smoked paprika

INSTRUCTIONS

1. Hard boil the eggs. I have found the best method is to start with the eggs at close to room temperature. Salt the water and bring to a boil. Gently drop them in. Turn the water down to a simmer. Cook for 11 minutes. Remove from the flame and quickly cold water bathe them. Let cool.

2. Peel and halve the eggs. Scoop out the yolks and put them in a small bowl. Set cooked egg whites aside on a plate.

3. In your small bowl, add all the ingredients to the egg yolks except the smoked paprika. Mash together with a fork until smooth.

4. With a spoon, fill the halved whites with the yolk mixture.

5. Sprinkle smoked paprika on top. Chill.

CRUSTLESS QUICHE

Makes 4 servings

Quiche is another great purpose for leftover ingredients. You can use almost any vegetable, but I would stay away from tomato as it contains too much water. I have made a quiche with shrimp, crab meat, broccoli, asparagus, peppers, low-fat mozzarella, low-fat swiss. The recipe below is my favorite. By using different herbs, you can create your own signature quiche. I make enough for reheating, as it is just as good the next day. Plate it with a tossed salad.

INGREDIENTS

Butter for greasing the baking dish
16 oz. sweet or spicy Italian chicken sausage
1 T olive oil
1 cup spinach
6 eggs
1 cup skim milk
1/4 tsp ground nutmeg
1/4 tsp salt
1/4 tsp fresh ground pepper
1/2 cup diced sweet onion

2 cups low-fat shredded cheese (Monterey Jack, cheddar, or four-cheese Mexican-style)

INSTRUCTIONS

1. Preheat the oven to 375 degrees Fahrenheit.
2. Grease an 8 x 8-inch baking dish, or a 8-inch-diameter pie pan.
3. Remove the sausage from the casing and sauté with the onion in olive oil. Continue to chop the sausage until it is very crumbly and thoroughly cooked.
4. Add the spinach and sauté for 15 seconds or so.
5. Whisk together eggs, milk, nutmeg, salt, pepper in a bowl.
6. Spread the sausage mixture on the bottom of the pan. Sprinkle the cheese evenly on top of the sausage. Pour the egg mixture over the top.
7. Place uncovered in the oven. Bake for 40 minutes.
8. Remove the dish from the oven and let it sit for 10 minutes to set.

OVERNIGHT OATS

Makes 2 hefty servings

The base for overnight oats is so simple to make. It is easy to add any flavor that you love. This is my go-to recipe. I make these in a large mason jar and use a coffee grinder to grind my nuts. You can store in the refrigerator for up to five days.

INGREDIENTS

1/2 cup uncooked oats
1/4 cup ground raw almonds (or other nuts)
1 cup almond milk (or other nut milk or nonfat dairy milk product of choice)
1/4 cup blueberries
1/4 cup raisins
Dash of cinnamon

INSTRUCTIONS

1. Mix the oats, almonds, cinnamon, raisins, and almond milk together and place them in a mason jar in the refrigerator overnight.
2. In the morning, dump the softened oats into a bowl and stir in the berries.

VARIATIONS

Substitute any kind of berries for the blueberries: strawberries, raspberries, blackberries.

Substitute apples or peaches.

Add a scoop of protein powder for a power punch—and increase with 1/4 more liquid if you do.

Substitute any kind of crumbled nuts for the almonds: walnuts or pecans work well.

SAUSAGE BEAN SOUP

Makes 8 servings

This is a great recipe to use your Instant Pot (or another pressure cooker), as the beans soften beautifully, and the time is significantly cut down to a cook time of about 30 minutes. This recipe offers two variations with completely different flavors of sausage made from either lamb or chicken. For a vegan option, it also can be made without meat altogether using no sausage and vegetable stock instead of bone broth.

INGREDIENTS

16 oz. dried lentils of any color, split peas of any color, or
    mixed beans
2 T olive oil
1/2 lb. chicken sausage or lamb sausage
1/2 cup each chopped red, green, yellow Bell peppers
1/2 cup chopped onion
1/2 cup chopped carrots
1 large clove garlic, chopped or pressed
1 tsp sage
1 tsp smoked paprika
1/4 tsp salt

1/4 tsp fresh ground pepper

1/4 tsp crushed dried red pepper

8 cups of organic chicken bone broth

15-1/2 oz. diced fire-roasted tomato, in juice from the can or
jar

Fat-free sour cream or nonfat Greek-style plain yogurt
(optional)

INSTRUCTIONS

1. Rinse the dried beans (see "Tip" below). While you are preparing your other ingredients, let the beans soak.
2. Heat 2 T olive oil in a good-sized soup pot.
3. Sauté the sausage, peppers, onion, carrots, garlic, and all the spices in the soup pot until the sausage is cooked.
4. Drain the beans and then stir them into the other ingredients.
5. Add the bone broth and diced tomatoes.
6. Cook on low for approximately 60 mins or until the beans are done, and the texture is creamy.

TIP

Let me give you a tip about preparing beans. I could not understand why my beans never thoroughly broke down to a nice creamy texture. Last year, my family moved, and I wanted to make my nice warming soup of lentils when it got chilly outside. I was kind of dreading the process, as in the past I would let the soup cool and then blend half of it to get the creamy texture I desired. But to my surprise, the soup turned out creamy with such great texture on its own. I had done nothing different except that the water I'd had in my previous house was "city water," which had a lot of minerals and calcium in it and had obviously gone through a process of decontamination. My new home has well water, which is soft. So, if you have hard water, I suggest that you rinse and soak your beans in store-bought spring water to get a creamier result.

VARIATIONS

Vegan option. Leave out the sausage and substitute the quantity with a mixture of your choice. I suggest adding celery, kale, and turnips Substitute vegetable broth for bone broth.

Add a dollop of fat-free sour cream or plain nonfat Greek-style yogurt to each serving.

CAESAR SALAD

Makes 4 dinner servings and 6 servings as a side dish

Caesar salad can be used as a side dish or as a full meal. I make the dressing ahead of time and what I don't use I freeze. In the summertime I make a point of growing romaine lettuce in my garden. The taste of fresh picked lettuce is remarkably different then store bought. I hope you all get to experience growing a garden.

INGREDIENTS
3/4 cup olive oil
3 T fresh-squeezed lemon juice
1 large clove garlic, chopped or pressed
1/2 cup grated parmesan cheese
1/4 tsp salt
1/4 tsp ground black pepper
1 large head romaine lettuce, washed

INSTRUCTIONS

1. For the dressing: In a jar or shaker, combine all the ingredients except the romaine. Shake very well.
2. Break apart the lettuce leaves into bite-sized pieces.
3. Pour the dressing over the lettuce and toss.

VARIATIONS

Lay anchovy fillets on top of your salad or chop the anchovy into small pieces and add to the dressing.

Top the salad with shaved parmesan. Use a vegetable peeler to shave from a block of cheese.

Top with slices of grilled chicken.

PORTOBELLO MUSHROOM PIZZA

Makes 8 servings

I call this "pizza," although we all know there is nothing like the real thing. If you're willing to give this a try and keep an open mind, you may be surprised! You can add many healthy toppings and still be on track with your weight loss. Some of the ones I like to use are garlic, spinach, ground meat (cook it first!), and olives.

I have discovered that using full-fat mozzarella makes the end result very watery. Therefore, I use low-fat mozzarella.

If you are baking, preheat the oven to 325 degrees.

You may also use a grill.

Serve with a tossed salad on the side.

INGREDIENTS

1 large portobello mushroom per person
Olive oil
Tomato sauce
Low fat shredded mozzarella
Any toppings of your choice

INSTRUCTIONS

1. Lightly rinse and clean the mushrooms with a soft potato brush. Pat dry. Gently remove the cores.
2. Lightly brush the bottom of each mushroom with olive oil.
3. If you are using chopped meat, spread the cooked meat in the cup of the mushroom first, before sauce or other toppings.
4. Spread enough tomato sauce in the cup of the mushroom to cover.
5. Cover the tomato sauce with cheese.
6. Sprinkle your toppings or toppings of choice over the cheese.
7. Place the mushrooms on a baking pan and place in the oven on the middle rack or on the grill. Roast until the mushrooms are tender.

FIRE-ROASTED TOMATO CHICKEN WITH RICE

Makes 4 servings

This chicken dish can be an entire meal. If you want to make this a one pot meal, don't make the rice as I suggested. Simply add yams to the chicken. This is what I call a warming meal. It is like a Chicken Soup for the Soul® type of thing. It's simple and quick comfort food.

INGREDIENTS

4 plump chicken breasts

2 T olive oil

1 large clove garlic, diced or pressed

Salt and pepper, to taste

1 T dried Italian seasoning (or any combination of dried basil, marjoram, oregano, rosemary, thyme)

15-1/2 oz. diced fire-roasted tomatoes, with juice from the can or jar

1/2 cup chopped fresh Bell peppers (green, red, orange, yellow, or multicolored)

1/2 cup chopped onion

4 cups brown rice, cooked (optional)

2 medium yams cut into 2-inch squares (optional)

INSTRUCTIONS

1. Check the cooking time on your brown rice and plan accordingly. The chicken should take approximately 30 minutes to cook.

2. Cut the chicken breasts into 2- to 3-inch chunks.

3. In a large skillet, sauté the chicken chunks in the olive oil until browned, seasoning them with garlic, salt, pepper, and Italian seasoning.

4. Add the Bell peppers and onions (add yams if you are using this option) and sauté until slightly cooked. Add the diced tomatoes with juice.

5. Simmer covered over a low flame for approximately 45 minutes, or until the chicken is tender.

6. Serve over a bed of brown rice.

STIR FRY

Makes 4 servings

When I have lots of vegetables that need to be used up soon, I either make soup or stir fry. I use almost any kind of vegetable for stir fry. I may have one sweet potato to add or a spare carrot or onion. Maybe some green beans or some leftover rice that I don't know what to do with. By the end, I have filled my entire wok, thinking I will have some leftovers for lunch—although that rarely happens because I usually gobble it all up. Here is the recipe that I often use. Feel free to experiment and make it your own! If you don't have a wok with high sides, a large skillet will do. This tastes great served over brown rice or wild rice.

INGREDIENTS

3 T sesame oil, divided
3 T freshly grated or ground ginger
3 T. soy sauce
1 lb. boneless chicken cut in bite-sized pieces
Large clove garlic, sliced thinly
1 cup carrots, chopped
1 cup broccoli, chopped
1 cup cauliflower, chopped

1 cup red cabbage, chopped

1 cup bok choy, chopped

1/2 cup snap peas, chopped

1/2 cup yellow or green zucchini, chopped

Ground black pepper, to taste

4 cups cooked brown rice or wild rice (optional)

INSTRUCTIONS

1. In a wok or large skillet, heat 2 T of sesame oil.
2. Add the chicken, 1 T grated ginger or ginger powder, and 1 T soy sauce. Stir frequently with a wooden spoon. While it is cooking, chop your vegetables into bite-sized pieces.
3. Cook the chicken until it is cooked through and slightly brown on the sides, and then remove it from the wok.
4. Add 1 T sesame oil, 2 T soy sauce, and garlic slices to the hot wok.
5. Start to stir-fry the densest, longest-cooking vegetables first: the carrots, broccoli, and cauliflower. Give them a 5-minute or so head start. If you need more fluid, start by adding ¼ cup or a few T of water. Stir frequently with a wooden spoon.
6. Add the red cabbage, bok choy, and snap peas. Stir.
7. Add the zucchini. Stir.
8. Add 2 T grated ginger and pepper. Stir.
9. Add the chicken back in. Stir.

VARIATIONS

Substitute shrimp, pork, or beef for the chicken.

VEGETABLE LASAGNA

Makes 6–8 servings, the contents of a 9 x 13-inch casserole dish or baking pan

You can improvise this dish with spinach, broccoli, and whatever combination of vegetables you have on hand in your refrigerator. My suggestions are in the ingredient list below. It also uses a "cheese" made from soft tofu, which is deliciously creamy as well as high in protein.

INGREDIENTS

2 T extra-virgin olive oil
4 cloves garlic, diced or pressed
1 16-oz container of silken (soft) tofu
1-1/2 cups grated parmesan, divided
1/2 tsp nutmeg
1 T white pepper
2 T low-sodium soy sauce
1/2 pound spinach
1 cup broccoli, chopped into bite-sized pieces
1 cup cauliflower, chopped into bite-sized pieces
1 cup mushroom slices
1 red Bell pepper, diced
1 carrot, sliced in thin rounds

2 eggs

1 large eggplant

4 cups tomato sauce

2 T dried basil (or 4 T fresh basil, chopped finely)

INSTRUCTIONS

1. Preheat oven to 350 degrees Fahrenheit.
2. Heat olive oil and garlic in a large pot over medium flame. Simmer for two minutes.
3. Open the tofu and set it to drain in a colander.
4. Add spinach, broccoli, cauliflower, mushrooms, Bell pepper, and carrot to your large pot, stirring occasionally, and cooking for 8–10 minutes until the vegetables are cooked halfway through. Remove from heat.
5. In a large mixing bowl, combine drained tofu with nutmeg, soy sauce, white pepper, and 1/2 cup parmesan cheese. Blend with a fork or spoon until creamy.
6. Stir the cooked vegetables and eggs into the blended tofu mixture. Set aside.
7. Slice the eggplant about 1/4-inch thick. Lightly salt it on both sides and let sit for 15 minutes or so. This will draw out the moisture. Pat both sides with paper towel.
8. To prepare your lasagna layers, go in the following order:
   - 1-1/3 cups tomato sauce on the bottom of the pan
   - layer of eggplant
   - 1/2 of the vegetable-tofu mixture
   - layer of eggplant

- 1-1/3 cups of tomato sauce. Sprinkle evenly with the basil.
- The rest of the vegetable tofu mixture
- layer of eggplant
- The rest of the tomato sauce (1-1/3 cups)
- Sprinkle 1 cup grated parmesan evenly across the top

9. Bake uncovered in the oven on the middle shelf for 45–60 minutes, until the top is golden brown (be careful not to burn the cheese or to dry out the edges of the pasta).
10. Cool on top of the stove for 10 minutes before slicing.

BASIC OLIVE OIL AND VINEGAR DRESSING

Yields 1-1/4 cup (20 tablespoons)

INGREDIENTS

1 cup extra-virgin olive oil

¼ cup balsamic vinegar

1 tsp. salt

1 tsp fresh ground pepper

1 T powdered or fresh garlic

1 tsp. dried Italian seasoning (or any combination of dried basil, marjoram, oregano, rosemary, thyme)

INSTRUCTIONS

1. Place all the ingredients in a mason jar or a sealed glass jar.
2. Shake well.
3. Use as needed. Store in a cool place.

Tips for Food and Beverage Choices During This Program

Some healthy living tips for food and drinks are:

- Replace sugary drinks with teas, such as chilled passion fruit tea, hot herbal teas or lemon water.
- Drink coffee in moderation. If you want to drink coffee, I suggest no more than two to four cups a day. No fake creamers and no sugar added.
- Eat plain yogurt. And remember, vanilla yogurt is *not plain* yogurt. Just because it is white does not mean there is no sugar added.
- Make your own dressing for salad with garlic, olive oil, balsamic vinegar, basil, oregano and lemon.
- Mix fresh fruit and nuts in yogurt or a hot cereal.
- Buy sugar-free frozen berries and make a smoothie with yogurt or thaw them out the night before and put them in hot cereal.
- Eat a handful of nuts before going out to dinner. This will help curb your appetite. Nuts are to be plain, unsalted. The label should say nuts. No oil.
- Plan ahead always carry a healthy snack.
- Keep it simple. Use my recipes and also go to the internet and find some good low-fat, sugar-free healthy meals. Crock pots or Insta pots are great for those who don't have time to cook themselves. Make enough for lunch the next day.

Some Simple Meal Ideas for Breakfast, Snacks, Lunch, Dinner

My clients always want to know what I eat every day. For starters, I must admit that I am not perfect, so don't look in my shopping cart! If I decide that I want chocolate ice cream or some warm bread with butter, I will think it through first to decide if it is really worth it. Then that bread had better be spectacular and the ice cream of the highest quality. You will never see me eat cake from a mix or store-bought cookies. If I do happen to indulge, I make sure to enjoy every bite, as it is a special event. I don't make an issue if I feel that what I consumed was not the healthiest choice. The key here is to immediately get back on track with what you're eating. I also will do a little extra exercise the next day. Maybe my walk will be a little longer or I will hike the trail with the big hill, and I'll do a little more intense weight-training workout. The idea is balance! Using myself as an example, here are a few ideas of what you could eat every day.

Breakfast

- Plain low-fat yogurt with fruit and nuts
- 2 scrambled eggs with lots of vegetables and 1 piece of fruit
- Overnight oats

Mornings Snacks

- 1 hard-boiled egg and 1 piece of fruit
- 1 T peanut butter on apple slices
- A smoothie with low-fat plain yogurt, frozen strawberries, and almond milk

Lunches

- A large salad made with homemade Basic Olive Oil and Vinegar Dressing (see page 133) with protein (beans, feta, chicken)
- Grilled chicken and/or vegetables
- Leftovers from the previous night's dinner

Afternoon Snacks

- Hummus and raw vegetables
- 100 calories of nuts and a hard-boiled egg
- A piece of fruit and a hard-boiled egg

Dinners

Dinner is always a meal that includes both a protein and some vegetables. If I am feeling hungry, then I add rice or a yam to my plate. Meals I also suggest are:

- Chicken and an abundance of vegetables.
- Hearty homemade soup, like Sausage Bean Soup (see page 118)

- Lean red meat and a large salad made with Basic Olive Oil and Vinegar Dressing (see page xxx)

YOUR VIBE IS YOUR TRIBE

At least four weeks have gone by. You have gotten a glimpse of your destination. Naturally you are going to encounter some rough seas. That is LIFE! Not every day will be all sweet berries and sugar-free whipped cream. You will encounter setbacks. Your focal point is the horizon ahead of you, a place of personal strength and vibrant health.

Here you are with your navigational chart in hand, the captain of your boat, steering clear of negative people and situations that will drag you down and the type of conditions that might send you back to where you were.

It doesn't matter if you're an elite athlete, a practiced guru, a weekend warrior, or this is the first time you've put on a **real** pair of workout sneakers. Everyone, and I mean *everyone* has to push the reset button and start over on a regular basis. What matters is that you don't let too many Mondays go by without taking action. What matters is that you picked up this book and began to follow the principles. What matters is that you know in your *heart* that *your* true north is not where you *were* but where you are *going*. True north is the place where the tribe that is going to love and support you wait with open arms. True north is the place where good health and a vibrant life awaits you. This is it! This is life, my fearless captain!

ACKNOWLEDGMENTS

There are so many people and experiences that contributed to me, here, at this point. Every day I learn something new that I am thankful for. I would not have been able to put my knowledge and experiences into words without my editor Stephanie Gunning's unwavering patience and intuitive ability to understand what I was trying to portray and her immense knowledge of her profession.

I want to thank Sean. Thank you for being patient. Thank you for understanding my extreme lack of technical skills and straightening out the computer disasters I created while trying to write this book. Thank you for teaching me that pushing random keys on the laptop won't get me a positive result. Mostly thank you for loving the high desert of Arizona as much as I do.

Thank you to photographer Javier Vargas and model Shannon Rose Corbitt, and cover designer Gus Yoo.

NOTES

Week One

1. Mayo Clinic staff. "Type 2 Diabetes," MayoClinic.org (accessed December 6, 2019), https://www.mayoclinic.org/diseases-conditions/type-2-diabetes/symptoms-causes/syc-20351193.
2. Andrew Weil. "Diet Soda Downside?" DrWeil.com (April 20, 2012) https://www.drweil.com/diet-nutrition/diets-weight-loss/diet-soda-downside.
3. Mehmet Oz. AZQuotes.com.
4. Anne Harding. "Downing diet soda tied to risk of premature birth," Reuters (June 30, 2010), https://www.reuters.com/article/us-diet-soda/downing-diet-soda-tied-to-risk-of-premature-birth-idUSTRE66M4AF20100723.
5. Robert H. Shmerling. "Sweeteners: Time to rethink your choices?" Harvard Health Blog/Harvard Medical School (February 22, 2019), https://www.health.harvard.edu/blog/sweeteners-time-to-rethink-your-choices-2019022215967.
6. News release. "UM Study Finds Possible Link Between Diet Soda and Vascular Risks," University of Miami. Miller School of Medicine (February 3, 2012),

http://med.miami.edu/news/um-study-find-possible-link-between-diet-soda-and-vascular-risks.

7. Vincent Martin. "Can aspartame trigger headaches?" Cincinnati Enquirer (July 24, 2016), https://www.cincinnati.com/story/sponsor-story/uc-health/2016/07/24/uc-health-headaches-sweeteners-aspartame-triggers/87076172.

8. Brett Molina. "Artificial sweeteners can still lead to obesity and diabetes, study claims," USA Today (April 23, 2018), https://www.usatoday.com/story/news/nation-now/2018/04/23/artificial-sweeteners-can-still-lead-obesity-and-diabetes-study-claims/541351002.

Week Two

1. "Bleached VS. Unbleached Flour," Organics.org (September 19, 2018), https://www.organics.org/bleached-vs-unbleached-flour.

2. "Topical Acne Products Can Cause Dangerous Side Effects," U.S. Food and Drug Administration (accessed December 6, 2019), https://www.fda.gov/consumers/consumer-updates/topical-acne-products-can-cause-dangerous-side-effects.

3. Luke Yoquinto. "The Truth about Potassium Bromate," LiveScience.com (May, 2013), https://www.livescience.com/36206-truth-potassium-bromate-food-additive.html. Also see "Consumer Group Calls for Ban on 'Flour Improver' Potassium Bromate Termed a Cancer Threat,"

Center for Science in the Public Interest (July 19, 1999), https://cspinet.org/new/bromate.html.

4. Andrew Weil. "A Carcinogen in Your Bread," DrWeil.com (July 16, 2012), https://www.drweil.com/diet-nutrition/food-safety/a-carcinogen-in-your-bread.

5. "Pure Food and Drug Act," Britannica.com (accessed November 29, 2019). Also see "Pure Food and Drug Act," Wikipedia.org (accessed November 29, 2019).

6. Deborah Blum. *The Poison Squad: One Chemist's Single-Minded Crusade for Food Safety at the Turn of the Twentieth Century* (New York: Penguin Press, 2018).

7. Alina Bradford. LiveScience "What Is the Hygiene Hypothesis?" LiveScience.com (March 17, 2016), https://www.livescience.com/54078-hygiene-hypothesis.html. Also see "Dr. Joseph Murray: Celiac Disease. A 'Best Of' show," Mayo Clinic Medical Edge Weekend podcast (November 26, 2011), https://newsnetwork.mayoclinic.org/discussion/dr-joseph-murray-celiac-disease-a-best-of-show.

8. William Davis. *Wheat Belly: Lose the Wheat, Lose the Weight, and Find Your Path Back to Health* (New York: Rodale, 2011), p. 77.

9. Ibid.

10. Stephanie Seneff. "Glyphosate Toxicity, Lowering Cholesterol and Getting Off Statins: Episode 238," Dave Asprey podcast (accessed December 6, 2019), https://blog.daveasprey.com/dr-stephanie-seneff-

glyphosate-toxicity-lower-cholesterol-naturally-get-off-
statins-238.

11. Leah Zerbe. "How Much Toxic Roundup Are You
Eating?" *Good Housekeeping* (March 13, 2017),
https://www.goodhousekeeping.com/health/diet-
nutrition/a20706601/how-much-toxic-roundup-are-you-
eating.

12. Tina Bellon. "In Roundup case, judge cuts $2 billion
verdict against Bayer to $86 million," Reuters (July 25,
2019), https://www.reuters.com/article/us-bayer-
glyphosate-lawsuit/in-roundup-case-u-s-judge-cuts-2-
billion-verdict-against-bayer-to-86-million-
idUSKCN1UL03G.

13. "Where are GMO crops and animals approved and
banned?" GNO FAQs/Genetic Literacy Project (accessed
December 6, 2019), https://gmo.geneticliteracyproject.
org/FAQ/where-are-gmos-grown-and-banned.

Week Three

1. Bill W. *Alcoholics Anonymous: The Big Book* (1939).

2. "Atherosclerosis," American Heart Association (accessed
December 6, 2019), https://www.heart.org/en/health-
topics/cholesterol/about-cholesterol/ atherosclerosis.

3. "Trans Fat," American Heart Association (accessed
December 6, 2019), https://www.heart.org/en/healthy-
living/healthy-eating/eat-smart/fats/trans-fat.

4. "Trans Fats Tied to Colorectal Polyps," Fight Colorectal Cancer (September 2, 2008), https://fightcolorectal cancer.org/blog/trans_fats_tied_to_colorectal_polyps.

5. "Trans Fats May Increase Risk," Breastcancer.org (accessed December 6, 2019), https://www.breastcancer.org/ research-news/20080411b.

6. "Final Determination Regarding Partially Hydrogenated Oils (Removing Trans Fat)," U.S. Food and Drug Administration (May 18, 2018), https://www.fda.gov/food/ food- additives-petitions/ final-determination-regarding-partially-hydrogenated-oils-removing-trans-fat.

Week Four

1. Betty Kovacs Harbolic. "Alcohol and Nutrition," MedicineNet.com (accessed November 11, 2019), https://www.medicinenet.com/alcohol_and_nutrition/art icle.htm#what_is_alcohol.

2. Ibid.

3. Tony Robbins. Tweet 10:10 AM Aug 28, 2015.

INDEX OF EXERCISES

INDEX OF RECIPES

DO YOU NEED MORE SUPPORT?

I would love to hear from you!

Hit me up on:

My website: www.StartThisMonday.life

Facebook: https://www.facebook.com/Starting-This-Monday-344564913052453/

Instagram: www.instagram.com/StartingThisMonday

ABOUT THE AUTHOR

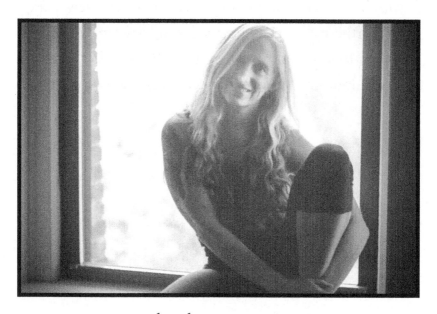

Photo by Jenna Lorenz

Patti Vanacore is a highly respected certified personal
fitness trainer and reiki master teacher who has devoted her
life to coaching people on the path to wellness. She has
helped hundreds of people attain their goals physically and
emotionally. While raising her children, she got
accreditation from the American Council on Exercise and
learned the art of balancing work, friends, fitness, and
fun. Over a successful thirty-year career, she has earned
recognition for incorporating many different types of
exercise into her work with her clients, including

kickboxing, martial arts, weight training, facilitated stretching, yoga, and reiki. She also possesses a vast knowledge of nutrition. Patti loves to be outdoors hiking with her friends and her dogs in New Jersey, New York, and Northern Arizona. She resides in New Jersey with her long-time significant other. In addition to her three children, she has five grandchildren and two dogs.

Made in the USA
Middletown, DE
23 January 2020

83625964R00099